Mastering Communication in Dentistry

Mastering Communication in Dentistry

The Secret to Long-term Patient Retention

Dr Milisha Chotai

Copyright © 2016 Dr Milisha Chotai
All rights reserved.

ISBN: 1537604597
ISBN 13: 9781537604596

Acknowledgements

I would like to dedicate this book to my husband, soul mate and best friend, Stefan. This book would never have been possible without his encouragement and support.

I would like to thank my parents for always believing in me and for introducing dentistry to me. I would also like to thank my family, colleagues and friends (especially Karen and Jo) for their constant encouragement throughout this process.

"Great Communication is a Skill, not an Accident"

-Dr Milisha Chotai-

Contents

Foreword xi
An Overview of Communication xv

Part I   Self-Awareness 1
1   Perception 3
2   Confidence 6
3   Optimism, Laughter and Passion 12

Part II   Mastering Communication 17
1   Non-Verbal Communication 19
2   Listening 25
3   Preparing for the First Visit 29
4   The First Patient Interaction 33
5   Presentation of a Treatment Plan 38
6   Influencing Patients 49
7   Breaking Bad News 52
8   Communicating Fees 57
9   Cross-Cultural Communication 68

Part III The "Difficult" Patient 73
1 Self-Assessment 75
2 The Human Element 79
3 Habit-Changing Communication 85
4 Relationship Building 87
5 Anxious Patients 95
6 Angry Patients 103
7 When Things Go Wrong 107

Part IV Electronic Communication 111
1 Electronic Mail 113
2 Social Media 117
3 Influencing In Writing 120
4 Digital Emotions 122

Afterword 126
Bibliography and Further Reading 129
Index 133

Foreword

Interpersonal communication is a skill that is lost in translation in dental education. Without excellent communication skills, clinical abilities alone are only going to take you so far in your career and work life. You may have the best hands in the world, but they will remain unused if you do not connect with your patient. I have spent the last eight years practicing dentistry in two very different countries and have realized that the clinical part of dentistry—although very important—is not a deciding factor in retaining patients and keeping them happy. You may be highly efficient and be seeing thousands of patients, but have you ever considered whether all of your patients really like you? Do they remember you? Are you irreplaceable? Dentistry is about repeat business; therefore, we cannot afford to take patients for granted.

Who am I? Why am I writing this book? My name is Milisha, and I was born and raised in Sweden. From an early age I was introduced to dentistry by my father, who is also a dentist. When I was halfway through dental school, I asked my father, *"Are root canal treatments the most complex part of dentistry?"* He responded, *"Sometimes"*. I did not realize what this actually meant until 3 years later, when I was based in a private practice in England.

Before relocating to England, I worked in a Swedish government clinic that had a standardized price list. While there, I focused exclusively on developing my clinical skills. Swedes are not intimate people, nor are they expressive. The Swedish language may sometimes come across as harsh to a non-Swede; joking and having a laugh can be perceived as immature, and small talk is not essential. Patients simply visit the dental clinic, receive their treatment and go home. My experience practicing dentistry in England was completely different; I was expected to chat, smile, and be friendly and polite. Suddenly, I was in a position in which selling determined my earnings. Although I knew that I had the required skill set to provide quality dentistry, I was finding it difficult to communicate this information to patients; and as a result, I was not busy. When my lack of patients began to affect my clinical practice and income, I realized that I had to change. I purchased books on communication, but they all focused on selling and were written by people who were not dentists. I therefore turned to literature on human behaviour and the psychology of interpersonal relationships. That literature changed everything! I was busier, my earnings increased, and my patients liked me. I began to enjoy practicing dentistry, and my passion grew from there!

You too can improve your clinical practice by improving your communication skills so that you can deliver what your patients want and need. This book will teach you how to be irreplaceable by giving you the ability to make your patients feel special and happy. My wish is for each and every patient to recognize you as an excellent person and clinician because that is what you deserve. My aim is to inspire and share with you what I have learnt over the years and giving you the ability not only to enter any patient relationship with increased confidence and control but also to manage your patients in a manner that makes them rave about you to everybody they know. Just imagine spending your life doing what you love, with patients you like, who like you back!

This book is not intended to be an in-depth analysis; rather, it is short, light and straight to the point. The concepts in this book are timeless, allowing you to return to it whenever you need a refresher. It is meant to complement your daily practice. This book is from me to you—from one dentist to another. I hope you enjoy it!

An Overview of Communication

Communication is a multi-faceted process that always involves more than one person. It is considered to be successful when it receives the desired response or reaction. It is helpful to imagine a loop when considering the multi-faceted nature of communication. The messenger who is positioned at one end of the loop chooses appropriate verbal and non-verbal codes that accompanies their message. The message is then transmitted through the appropriate medium (voice, writing, face-face). The receiver who is at the other end of the loop will receive, decode and perceive the message. The message will only be accurately perceived if the receiver uses the same codes as the messenger. The receiver's feedback is the response or reaction which could be another signal or action.

Figure 1: The communication loop.

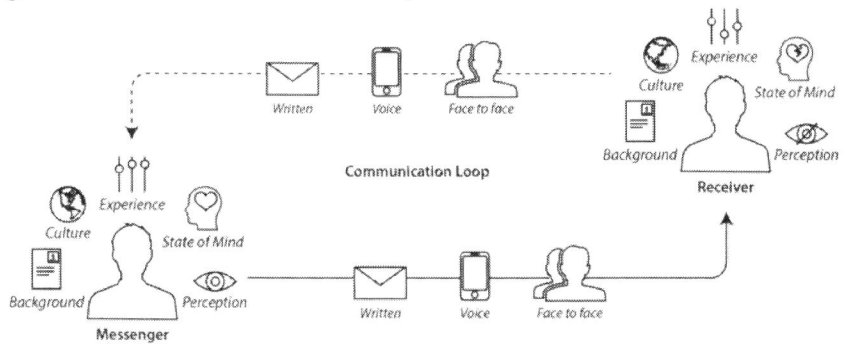

Part I

Self-Awareness

Your self-concept and how comfortable you are in your own skin will influence how you interact with the people around you. Dentists who understand themselves and accept who they are have the ability to connect with patients by seeing the world through their eyes. They do not worry about rejection and are less likely to make judgements. We have to therefore work on ourselves before we work on others; knowing and understanding yourself will make significant improvements in your interaction with your patients.

One

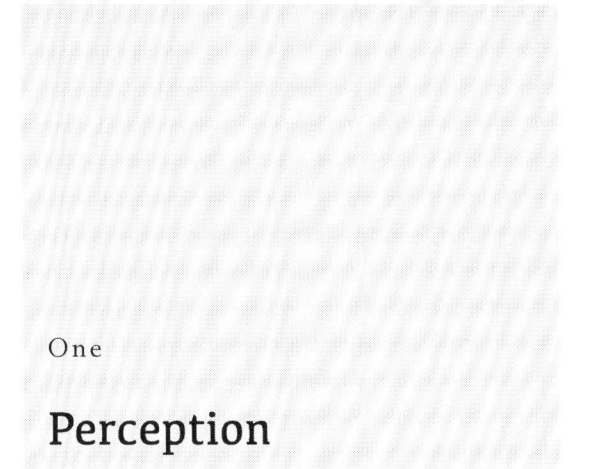

Perception

Perception is our ability to apply meaning to sensory information. The perception of words and behaviour is an unconscious process that is influenced by our state of mind, experiences, past, personality, beliefs, goals, and culture. It is the reason for both disagreements and agreements; it is why we readily get along with people who are similar to us and why we do not always see eye-to-eye with those who are different to us.

Recognizing perception as a limiting factor in your communication will enable you to not only accept that there are two sides to one story but that disagreements are not necessarily personal; but instead, they are a result of both differences in perception and people seeing the same truth with different set of lenses. At the end, it does not matter what you mean; what matters is how your patient perceives what you mean.

SELECTIVE HEARING
Mesgarani and Chang (2012) found that the representation of speech in the brain cortex does not reflect only external sounds; but instead, it also reflects what we perceive as interesting and important. This

means that your perception may influence what you hear. In dental practice, "selective hearing" is the reason for why you could miss vital information that your patient has disclosed, or the reason for why your patient could deny of having been informed of their treatment implications. Recognizing that selective hearing is not a shortcoming but a biological process will enable you to avoid conflicts when a patient tells you, *"That is not what I said"* or *"That is not what you said"*.

SELECTIVE MEMORY

Our self-perception and goals influence what information we choose to retain. Information that is more congruent with our existing personality, goals, needs and experience is more likely to be retained in memory than information that is less congruent with our beliefs. Therefore, patients are more likely to remember information they can relate to and that goes in line with their beliefs, wants and needs. This also explains why your patient might sometimes twist and interpret information presented by you to suit their liking and needs.

REJECTION AND SELF-PERCEPTION

As highly social animals, we strive for acceptance, which is why we do not feel comfortable when we hear the word "no". Rejection is automatically translated into a lack of acceptance, which is inconsistent with our basic human needs. The impact of rejection is both psychological and physiological. A study at the University of Michigan found that rejection triggers and involves the same neural pathways that are activated when we experience severe pain.

Self-perception plays a vital role in how we cope with rejection and influences the frequency of rejections that we encounter. Rejections are more common amongst people who expect them than among people who are positive and do not expect to be rejected. Guy Winch, a clinical psychologist, states that rejection is responsible for only 50% of our reactions, with the other 50% based on our self-perception. People with low self-esteem tend to be more sensitive to rejection. In response, they become preoccupied with their "hurt feelings", thus increasing the risk of further rejection. This process can become a vicious circle for the rejection-sensitive person. For example, a patient who is rejecting your proposed treatment plan. If you are too busy thinking about yourself and your feelings, you are less likely to empathize with your patient. As a result, the patient will not change his or her mind and accept the treatment plan.

Awareness of how you perceive yourself will enable you to understand your role in the rejection process. Rejection of your treatment plans, your fees or even you as a person can all be prevented if you display confident body language and work on not becoming pre-occupied with yourself as a result of failing to gain acceptance.

Two

Confidence

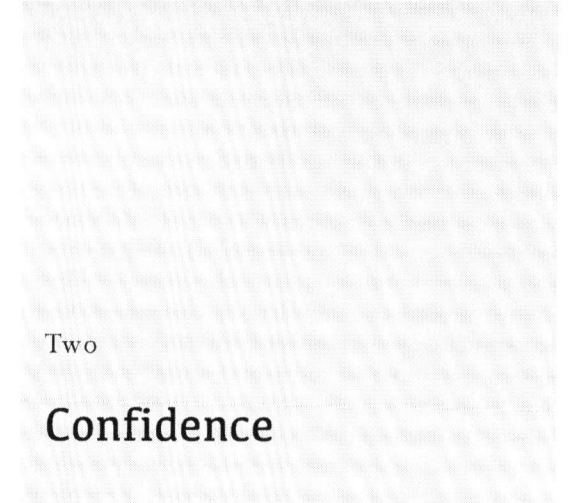

Have you ever socialized with a person who does not believe in him- or herself and constantly needs validation? People are more likely to enjoy the company of a confident person who does not need constant validation. In a dental situation, patients come to you to receive care. The last thing they want is to feel that they have to take care of you or convince you of your abilities.

Confidence is a state of mind that arises from believing in your own ability to achieve and not being afraid of failing. A lack of confidence will negatively affect how your patient perceives you and may make it difficult for him or her to trust you. As a result, the patient might attempt to take charge of the treatment, sometimes even convincing you to perform procedures against your recommendations.

Confident people do not have to boast about themselves; their belief in themselves resonates in everything they say and do. Their non-verbal behaviour speaks for them. You must resonate confidence if you want to gain your patients' trust. According to the great American dancer Martha Graham, "The body never lies". A lack of confidence is more clearly revealed through non-verbal communication than through words. Your patient will sense that "something is off" if your unconfident non-verbal communication fails to align with your words.

Table 1: Habits that communicate a lack of confidence.

HABITS THAT COMMUNICATE A LACK OF CONFIDENCE
• Speaking over patients • Being short tempered • Inability to accept being wrong • Boasting • The need to be in focus • Requiring constant validation • Being timid • Not making eye contact • Fidgeting

Table 2: Habits that communicate confidence.

HABITS THAT COMMUNICATE CONFIDENCE
• Resting your eyes on your patient before looking away • Taking initiative to make eye contact • Using hand gestures to end sentences • Being calm and smiling • Conveying a polished professional appearance • Standing/sitting up tall

I have great news for you! Developing confidence is possible, and if you are proactive, it does not have to take a long time. Here are some great techniques for building your confidence:

1. **Role-play.** Imagine a confident, fantastic you, and play that role. How would you look? How would you speak? What would you say? What would your body language be like? Play the role until the confident behaviour becomes automatic. Your mind-set will follow. Confident body language includes making eye contact, smiling lightly, sitting up straight and not fidgeting.
2. **Model someone whom you admire.** Pick a person that you look up to and study their behaviour. How do they speak and interact with people? Practice and model these behaviours.
3. **Surround yourself with a solid and positive support system.** I have two positive and enthusiastic nurses, Jo and

Karen, who believe in me and trust me. Patients see their trust in me as reassuring; as a result, they are more likely to trust me.

4. **Find a mentor whom you admire.** Sometimes you just need a push to believe in yourself. Positive feedback from a mentor whom you admire is very powerful because you automatically trust his or her opinion. I look up to my mentor, Jonathon, and everything that he has achieved. Knowing that your mentor believes in you will inspire confidence in yourself.
5. **Further your knowledge in your chosen field.** Engage in continuous professional development courses. The letters behind your name testify to what you know. Reading one hour a day in your chosen field will also boost your knowledge, and you will be far ahead of your competitors. In turn, becoming an expert will stimulate your confidence.
6. **Groom yourself!** Who does not feel amazing after visiting the hairdresser or wearing a new dress/suit? Make a point of always looking your best. I feel much more confident when I make an effort with my appearance. Indeed, I always spend longer on my appearance when I will be presenting extensive treatment plans or when I anticipate experiencing a stressful situation during the day. It makes me feel great that I look good, and my confidence is boosted.
7. **Don't be afraid of failing.** Norman Vincent Peale said, "When God wants to send you a gift, he wraps it up in a problem". Although problems are a pain, if you look closely to determine why they have occurred, you will definitely find your gift. See the situation for what it is. No one is going to die! Get

used to resistance; every failure will bring you closer to success if approached in the correct manner.

8. **Practice the hero pose.** It works every time. Do the following before a stressful event: stand up with your back straight and feet hip width apart, hands on hips and chest out. Stand like that for 60 seconds, and you will immediately feel like a superhero who can survive anything.

9. **Lucky charms.** Have you ever thought about why it is difficult to throw away objects for which you have no need? The particular object has a memory or an emotion attached to it and triggers a subconscious process that makes you feel something positive. When I bought my dental practice, I purchased a Chopard Hamsa bracelet. The bracelet is made of white gold with a floating diamond in the middle. The bracelet retails at £1,200, and when I first saw it, it appeared to be an unattainable luxury that I could do without because there were better and more important things in which to invest my hard-earned money. I decided to save for a year, after which I would buy it for myself. I wear my bracelet every time I am about to encounter a situation that makes me nervous. The bracelet signifies that nothing is impossible if I work hard. Wearing this bracelet brings back memories of a spring morning when I went to Bond Street in London and the doorman opened the Chopard boutique's door for me. I sat next to the mahogany desk and watched as the sales assistant wrapped up my bracelet. The bracelet brings back clear memories of what it felt like to walk down Bond Street carrying a Chopard bag: the sweet feeling of success.

Of course, there are many other ways of building confidence; you have to find the one that works for you. Just remember the importance of having confidence because without it, neither patients nor the other people around you will judge you fairly.

Three

Optimism, Laughter and Passion

OPTIMISM

Being optimistic and happy is very important for both success and sanity. Feeling unhappy will set you back seriously both at work and in life. Imagine if I started this book by quoting suicide rates for dentists and the new high in dental malpractice litigation. Would you want to continue reading this book? Would it make you excited? Would it be worth spending precious time reading something that makes you miserable? When I think about optimism and positive people, I naturally think of my husband, Stefan, who always has a smile on his face. He smiles when he is awake, and he smiles when he is asleep. His life is all about being happy, and I cannot begin to tell you how contagious this attitude is. Optimism will also make your patients feel hopeful, happy and at ease.

Conversely, pessimism will make your patients feel sad, angry and hopeless. Like optimism, pessimism is a contagious trait; you can upset people by being pessimistic. I have a friend who is always negative. Speaking to her for 15 minutes is exhausting! I leave the conversation feeling completely drained and anxious. As a result, I avoid speaking to her more often than necessary.

Like confidence, optimism is both a strength and a skill; you have to practice it to master it. Try being positive for one day and see how good you feel at the end of that day. I will bet you a pair of Jimmy Choos that people around you will be jolly as a result and that you will feel great! The more optimism you radiate, the more you receive in return and the more people want to be around you. This includes your patients. Why would your patients not want to be treated by you when you are making them feel happy? Your optimism will induce a "feel-good factor", which is necessary if you are to have happy patients who purchase treatments and recommend you to their friends and family.

SMILING

Have you ever greeted someone with a wide smile and received a gloomy facial expression as a return? I haven't. Research shows that smiling is contagious and can make us appear attractive to others (Hatfield, 1992). Smiling also releases endorphins and fights stress (Seaward, 2009). Every time I see a patient, I switch on my smile as if I am seeing a good friend. This communicates that I am confident, relaxed and genuinely happy to see them. Such are the benefits of a smile!

LAUGHTER

Did you know that rats and dogs can laugh? Did you also know that laughing rats and dogs tend to surround themselves with fellow laughing rats and dogs? Human beings have this trait in common with rats and dogs; if we laugh a lot, we tend to want to surround ourselves with people who laugh with us. Like optimism and smiles, laughter is naturally contagious. This is why you will sometimes find yourself laughing at jokes at stand-up comedy shows.

Laughter is not only a response to jokes but also a form of communication that shows people that we like and understand them. Robert

Provine, a psychologist from the University of Maryland, found that we laugh the most when talking to our friends. Making a patient laugh or laughing with them establishes a friendly connection. I strongly believe that grumpy dentists will have grumpy co-workers and grumpy patients. The opposite is true for a dentist who laughs a lot. Hopefully, these are enough reasons why you should laugh a bit!

PASSION

Do you know why you do what you do? If you don't, it is time for some quality soul-searching. To communicate passion, you need to find what makes you happy. Dentistry is unlikely to make a patient excited and happy if it does not do the same for you. You will excel at whatever makes you happy, and you will remain average or below average at whatever does not make you happy and ignite that fire in you. Life is a gift, and time is limited. Time is an asset that once wasted will never return to you. Why would you spend your precious time doing anything other than your favourite thing in the world? It is logical to conclude that the more passion we have for something, the more time we will spend doing it and the better we will be at it. Anyone who knows me knows that I love what I do and that I am very passionate about it. How? It resonates through me! I love my job, and I love waking up in the morning to go to work. I miss work when I am away on holidays, and I always take some work-related reading with me when I go away. I take time off to spend quality time with my husband, not to be away from dentistry. I make sure I tell patients how much I love my job; as a result, they seem to enjoy their dental experience more than they would otherwise. No one wants to be around miserable Joe who hates what he does.

Assuming that you are passionate, below are some methods of communicating your passion.

- **Get excited!** Tell your patients how excited you are about your dental tools. Tell them what they do, where you bought them and how much they cost. I once bought a very expensive piece of equipment instead of going to Canada for a holiday. I tell my patients about it every time I use it. They love hearing about it, first because they know that I am investing in expensive equipment for their benefit and second because it makes them laugh.
- **Surprise your patients with your excitement!** I once bought a fancy bur kit. I told the patient that he was the first one to have the pleasure of the kit and how fun it was going to be to use it. I immediately had this patient laughing and in a good mood.
- **Report what you learnt** from courses or conferences. Patients love to hear that you keep current with the latest advances in your field. These reports show that you enjoy what you do.
- **Your qualifications are a testimony of your passion.** Tell your patients about them. Tell them about your course work, and tell them about how much you enjoy working even though it might sometimes take over your life.

When I look back at those patients with whom I have formed a connection, what they all have in common is that I have not only communicated my passion and optimism about dentistry but also laughed with them.

Part II

Mastering Communication

Dentistry is not about teeth; it is about people with teeth. People are creatures of emotions whose actions are guided by prejudice, fear, pride, and sometimes (rarely) logic. Communication is a means of accurately conveying what you think and mean. It can be divided into verbal and non-verbal forms that should align to communicate a single message to avoid misunderstandings.

One

Non-Verbal Communication

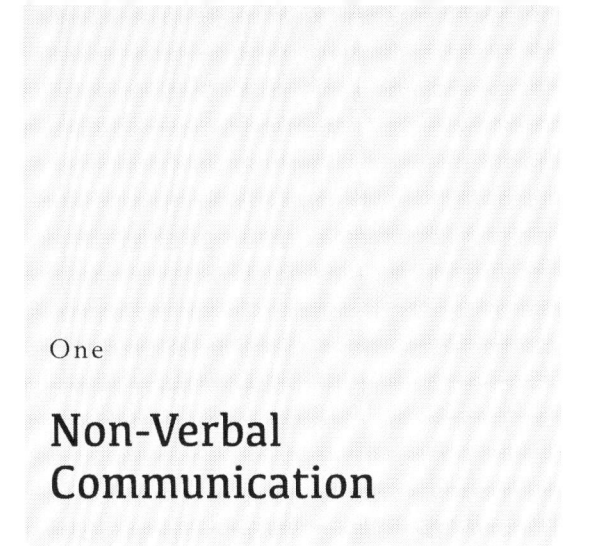

Non-verbal language refers to the wordless clues that give meaning to our spoken words.

It is innate and reflects our emotions, thoughts and intentions. Patients will search for non-verbal cues about what they should be feeling and thinking as you deliver the facts about their dental health. Inconsistencies between non-verbal and verbal communication can be perceived as a lack of genuineness and may result in patients questioning your true intentions. Having the ability to interpret your patients' non-verbal language will also enable you to tailor your delivery of information in a manner that suits their needs.

CONFLICTING COMMUNICATION

Conflict between verbal and non-verbal communication will always result in the recipient relying on the non-verbal communication. For example, telling your patient that you would like to help while avoiding eye contact and not smiling will send the message that your help is not genuine or that you dislike the patient. It is therefore essential that your non-verbal communication remains consistent with your verbal communication, thus relaying consistent messages.

EYE CONTACT
Facing the patient while maintaining eye contact conveys honesty, integrity and interest. The more you like someone, the more eye contact you will make. The more your eyes meet the patient's eyes, the more you will like each other. Looking straight into a patient's eyes is an alpha male trait and can promote defensive or aggressive behaviour. Moreover, it can be perceived as too intimate for a professional relationship. However, avoiding direct eye contact communicates unfriendliness and insecurity.

Balance is key; eye aversion (e.g., blinking) is an important technique in controlling and balancing the amount of eye contact during a conversation.

PERSONAL SPACE
Edward T. Hall, an American anthropologist who studies personal distance, writes that our brains cope with the invasion of personal space by dehumanizing other people. Dehumanization includes avoiding eye contact, maintaining a neutral facial expression and talking minimally. This explains why we tend to look at the floor or the walls when crammed into an elevator space rather than making eye contact with the surrounding people.

As dentists, we are constantly encroaching on our patients' personal space. Worse yet, there are no barriers to protect their personal space. Patients may become physically ill or uncooperative to regain a social distance that is more acceptable for strangers (the dentist) or non-intimate acquaintances (the dentist). You can prevent negative reactions by taking your time to get to know your patient at a social interpersonal distance of approximately one metre before invading their personal space.

POSTURE

Sitting at the same level as your patient will portray you as a caring and confident dentist. Standing to look down on your patient will make you look unsympathetic and controlling. Leaning backward and away from the patient may reflect a negative attitude of superiority. Leaning slightly forward will show that you are genuinely interested in what the patient has to say. Also keep in mind that your posture will influence how you feel. For example, you will feel more confident when sitting up straight than when slouching.

BODY MOVEMENTS

- **Hand gestures:** Pointing your hands or fingers may portray you as rude, condescending or confrontational. Frantically moving your hands as you speak will make you seem disorganized and can induce anxiety in your patient. Deception cues associated with hand gestures generally take the form of the hands digging into the cheeks and picking at fingernails. Fingers at the lips can represent shame, and touching your face can portray you as insecure. Keep your hands relaxed and visible to communicate honesty, confidence and calmness.
- **Head positioning:** Bringing your hand to your head will show that you are interested in your patient. Tilting your head to your hand will communicate boredom.
- **Leg positions:** Tense leg positions or fidgeting communicates deception or nervousness.

FACIAL EXPRESSIONS

Facial expressions are emotional and involuntary. They communicate the seven basic human emotions: anger, contempt, disgust, fear, happiness, sadness and surprise. According to Aaron Sell, a psychology professor at Griffiths University School of Criminology, expressions are cross-culturally universal. Indeed, congenitally blind children practice them without ever having seen them. Vivid facial expressions usually convey energy, enthusiasm and strong emotions. Angry facial expressions include a thinned lip, lowered brow and flared nostrils. Your facial expressions should match what you are trying to achieve with your words. A light smile and a neutral facial expression will communicate interest in your patient. Using vivid expressions will communicate passion, whereas neutral facial expressions when talking about what you do will communicate boredom.

The face is composed of 44 muscles, most of which remain unused throughout the day and thus stiffen and do not contribute to your facial expression. Frances Coles Jones, the author of *"How to WOW: Proven strategies for selling your brilliant self in any situation"*, writes about the importance of vivid facial expressions to make a long-lasting impression. She describes an exercise called the pumpkin/raisin face in which you first stretch your face out, widen your mouth and open your eyes as much as possible while sticking your tongue out as far as possible. Next, the face is made small as a raisin by pursing your mouth tightly, squeezing your eyes closed, sucking your cheeks in and furrowing your brows. Tense facial muscles limit the degree of facial expressions that we can make. Broadening the scope of your facial expressions will make your face more approachable and interesting. Your face will be more alive and expressive; as a result, you are more likely to catch the attention of the person to whom you are speaking.

PARA-LANGUAGE

Albert Mehrabian, a psychology professor, explains that our tone of voice (volume, emotion and emphasis on words) is responsible for approximately 35%-40% of our message. For example, speech that is shaky or slow will come across as lacking confidence. Patients will always rely on your para-language to determine the true meaning of your words.

- **Speed:** Speak in phrases that the patient can easily follow. Speaking too fast communicates fear, anger or impatience. Speaking too slow can reflect either sadness or a sense that your patient is inferior. Slowing one's speech when explaining a treatment plan is very useful for elderly and anxious patients. Tailor your speed to your patient.
- **Volume:** Speak at a normal conversational volume and emphasize key words.
- **Pitch:** A very high pitch conveys excitement, and a very low pitch will make you sound dull/depressed or boring. A medium to high pitch conveys happiness and is suitable both at the beginning of your conversation and when greeting your patient. A medium to low pitch is suitable for serious discussions. A high pitch when discussing serious issues could confuse your patient.

TOUCH

Touching your face signals that you need comfort and can portray you as insecure. In addition, be aware that your hands must be clean! Do not touch your teeth or mouth in front of the patient (I have seen some dentists do this). Politely touching the patient's shoulder is usually effective in communicating empathy, but make sure that you only do so once you have established a sense of familiarity. Touching a patient who sees you as a total stranger can be considered too intimate or threatening.

UNDIVIDED ATTENTION AND AFFIRMATION

Undivided attention accompanies listening to your patient. Your undivided attention will make patients feel important and will help them to develop trust in you. Patients will genuinely be interested in you if you are genuinely interested in them. The following techniques can be utilized to convey your undivided attention:

- Face the patient when speaking to him or her to show respect and appreciation.
- Nodding and smiling lightly will convey that you understand and would like your patient to continue speaking.
- Make intermittent eye contact.
- Do not multitask; let your nurse quietly do the typing in the background.
- Encourage your patient by asking open-ended questions.
- Eliminate background noise (radio, slamming instruments, open door, phone ringing).

DON'T OVERDO IT: YOU COULD LOOK STRANGE!

Non-verbal communication is innate and universal. Human beings thus have an innate ability to recognize unnatural body language, which is interpreted as strange and not genuine.

Two

Listening

Have you ever had a conversation with someone who is constantly interrupting you? It is likely to leave you feeling stressed, anxious and unimportant. If there is one communication skill that you need to master, it is the art of listening. This is the most important part of non-verbal communication. It is so important that I have dedicated a full chapter to it! A good listener will automatically be a great conversationalist, and your patients will love you if they can pour their hearts out to you, knowing that you are genuinely interested in what they have to say. People love themselves; they like to talk about themselves, and they find whatever they say to be the most interesting thing in the world. Being genuinely interested in what your patients have to say automatically results in your taking a genuine interest in them, making them feel desired and important. Being a good listener will also prevent misunderstandings and breakdowns in communication that could leave the patient feeling frustrated and angered.

LISTENING VERSUS HEARING

I am sure that you are familiar with the following situation, which occurs weekly in my house. I am talking to Stefan about something I find important while he is facing the TV and not responding. My perception is automatically that what I am saying is not important to Stefan. From Stefan's point of view, he is successfully multitasking by watching the news and listening to his wife. So I ask, "Why are you not listening?" He responds, "I am listening to you", and then he repeats what I have said to show me that he did indeed listen. Somehow, I remain unsatisfied because I feel that what I have said is unimportant to Stefan because he is not giving me his undivided attention. Stefan has been hearing, not listening. Listening is an attentive process that requires concentration and paying attention by analysing the meaning of words and observing nonverbal cues that accompany those words. Hearing, in contrast, is superficial communication in which words are not associated with meaning or emotion. A patient who does not feel attentively listened to will respond by repeating themselves. This is a signal for you either to step up your listening skills or to communicate that you have listened and understood.

CHARACTERISTICS OF A POOR LISTENER

We cannot improve if we do not know what we are doing wrong. Poor listeners find that what they have to say is more important than what the other person is saying. They are usually impatient, and their mind is usually preoccupied with other things, making it difficult to focus. Poor listeners are more occupied with the answer than the question. For example, they will try to interrupt so that they can fill in the blanks or give unsolicited advice. They are usually looking for an opportunity to interrupt. They may have a need to be the focus, which is why they do not allow the spotlight to be taken away from them.

HOW TO LISTEN

BE QUIET
Mark Twain said, "If we were supposed to talk more than we listen, we would have two tongues and one ear". Listening is an extension of hearing. It involves being verbally attentive by understanding words. You are

attuned to what the patient volunteers to tell you. This cannot take place unless you are quiet. It is truly amazing how silence can make a patient open up. Just remaining quiet can be more powerful than any other tool to put your patient at ease. Do not interrupt when someone is talking. Do not act like you have something on your mind because this will only make your patient feel rushed and unimportant. Forget about everything that you want to say, and realize that the stage is not yours.

FOCUS
Forget about everything that is happening around you. Eliminate distractions and focus on your patient as if he or she is about to present some very important and ground-breaking news.

ENCOURAGE
Smile lightly and nod to encourage your patient to continue. This also shows understanding and agreement. Make intermittent eye contact (do not stare and do not look away).

UNDIVIDED ATTENTION AND UNCONDITIONAL POSITIVE REGARD
Do not fidget, pick your nails or look away; these activities will make you seem bored or distracted. Let the patient take the time to speak his or her mind. Some patients will need to pause to think; let them. Do not interrupt or finish their sentences for them. Unconditional positive regard for the patient to communicate his or her worries and concerns is key. Listen with your eyes; non-verbal cues can tell you when the patient has a question, when he or she wants to say something, and when he or she agrees or disagrees with you.

ANALYSE
Look at the patient's non-verbal cues and tone. Try to identify the hidden meaning behind his or her words.

EMPATHIZE AND ENCOURAGE

Put yourself in your patient's shoes. Understand from their perspective. Do not disagree, which can cause distress and conflict. Keep an open mind, and ask open-ended questions to show that you are interested.

SUMMARIZE

Ensure that the patient is finished before you summarize. Always ask, *"Is there anything else?"* if you are uncertain. I always tell patients that I would like to summarize to ensure that I have understood what the patient has said. This makes them feel important. They will also have the opportunity to add information that they forgot to mention.

MAKE WAY FOR A DIALOGUE

Before you know it, the summary of the monologue has usually turned into a dialogue. You are inviting a conversation based on patient's wants and needs. I can guarantee that you will be surprised by the amount of useful information that the patient will disclose as a result of your now excellent listening skills.

Three

Preparing for the First Visit

The benefits of prioritizing and spending time on the initial consultation are endless. The way you approach this appointment will set the tone for your future relationship with the patient. The well-known statement by Seth Godin, "Dig your well before you are thirsty", should be kept in mind when determining the quantity (time) and quality (attention) that you dedicate to the initial consultation. The ultimate goal is for the patient to trust that you are considering his or her best interests, to accept your recommendations and to experience treatment without major anxiety. Spending quality time laying the foundation for a positive relationship with your patient will also help you when things do not go according to plan (unfortunately, we cannot always predict the future). The trusting patient will understand you, not blame you. The patient will also feel comfortable telling you if he or she is unsatisfied with any aspect of your service, which in turn gives you the opportunity to put things right.

FIRST IMPRESSION

The patient will take 5 seconds to formulate a first impression of you as his or her future dentist. You will unfortunately not be judged on your excellent clinical skills or the fact that you are a great person.

Amy Cuddy, a Harvard Business School social psychologist, says that we form not one impression but two when we first meet a new person. The first impression is based on how trustworthy the person is, and the second impression is based on how confident the person is. Cuddy's research shows that these two traits constitute up to 90% of first impressions. Patients will judge you not only on your verbal and non-verbal communication but also on your personal attributes, including clothing, grooming and cleanliness (Rehman et al, 2005). You should speak clearly with intermittent eye contact, making sure that your handshake is not like a dead limb but is firm. Wear a clean and well-ironed outfit, which will communicate confidence and control.

ENVIRONMENT

The setting in which the patient receives care will affect treatment satisfaction. Factors such as decor, colour, furnishings, room temperature, and furniture arrangement can influence your patient's psychological and physiological attitudes towards dental care. Beautiful rooms (drapes, carpets, etc.) have been shown to produce feelings of pleasure, comfort and the desire to continue an activity (Basehart, 1975). Blue interiors signify security and comfort. Black and brown colours signify unhappiness and hostility. Yellow interiors signify cheerfulness and joyfulness (Basehart, 1975). Obstacles such as tables and desks between the dentist and the patient are likely to be interpreted as too formal and may make the patient feel uncomfortable. Sitting on the same side as your patient will place him or her at ease and will set the scene for a friendly discussion instead of a formal interview.

PERSONAL ATTRIBUTES

Taking care to look your best will not only make you feel great but also will make your patients feel great. They will be more likely to confide in you and be satisfied with you if you are dressed appropriately (Rehman et al, 2005). A clean and well-ironed outfit also indicates professionalism and hygiene. Appropriate attire and a smiling face is an unbeatable combination. A carefully dressed and prepped dentist will convey the message that the meeting is important, whereas the untidy dentist may be perceived as uncaring and uninterested. Name badges are generally preferred by patients, especially if you have a name that patients find difficult to remember. It has been found that less-acceptable items to patients generally include facial piercings, short tops, brightly dyed hair, training shoes, sandals, loose hair, skirts above the knee, long earrings, multiple rings, sleeveless tops, ties depicting cartoon characters or no tie at all (Lil and Wilkinson, 2005).

SCHEDULING THE APPOINTMENT

Ensure that you schedule the patient consultation at a suitable time—not when you anticipate running late, because this might communicate either that you are unreliable or that your planning is inadequate. Running late will also stress you, which will be reflected in your communication. You may miss out on important non-verbal cues from the patient and rush into encroaching on his or her personal space. Your hand gestures may be all over the place, and you may speak too quickly. If you are running late, make sure that you communicate that information to your patient through reception. Being kept in the dark about one's appointment is awful, especially because people have busy lives. Moreover, a lack of information can elevate anxiety levels amongst already anxious patients. Imagine an anxious patient who is waiting for his or her appointment, which has been delayed by more than ten minutes. The patient will wonder what has gone wrong to make you run late. Next, the patient will be rushed into the surgery room and is likely to have his or her personal space invaded by a frightening, unknown individual (you) in a foreign environment (dental surgery). It doesn't take a genius to recognize that this situation will not yield ideal results.

Four

The First Patient Interaction

IDENTIFY YOUR PATIENT'S EMOTIONAL STATE

This is where your now amazing non-verbal communication skills will come to use. Pay attention to how the patient walks in. Hunched up and terrified? Strolling in with a smile? Rushing in with a stack of papers? All of these behaviours will give you a cue about how to best start the conversation. Ask the patient to sit in the dental chair and observe the reaction. Observe the patient's facial expression and body language. Open the conversation by saying, *"Today, we are seeing you for a dental examination"*. Pause to provide a window for the patient to speak. Patients will either happily agree, or they will feel encouraged to open up about themselves. Some patients may even say that they do not want a check-up. By asking the question, you are giving the patient control of the appointment. Accept that most patients do not enjoy going to the dentist. Although not all such patients are anxious, most are uncomfortable. Remember the personal space theory (Part 1, chapter 1): we are strangers encroaching on the patient's personal space. For that reason, it would be odd for the patient not to be hesitant. You must let the patient decide when he or she is ready to let you conduct the examination. A good way is to simply ask the question, *"Is it ok for me to have a look at your teeth?*" This will ensure that you are not forcing yourself into their personal space.

IT IS ALL ABOUT THE PATIENT

Accept that this is a one-man show—not yours, but the patient's! This appointment is all about making your patient feel special. Indicate that you want the patient to feel good about him- or herself and say that you are not judging. Make the patient feel important by giving him or her honest appreciation and a compliment. Women love to be complimented on their hair, nails and shoes. Men like to be complimented on their hair and shoes or anything else that you may find worthy of a compliment. Make sure that your compliment is genuine.

ENCOURAGING THE PATIENT TO OPEN UP

Patients rarely reveal their histories without encouragement. I have occasionally started treatment and suddenly realized that my patient was anxious. At such times, I would have benefitted from probing deeper while taking the patient's history.

Table 3: How to get the patient to open up.

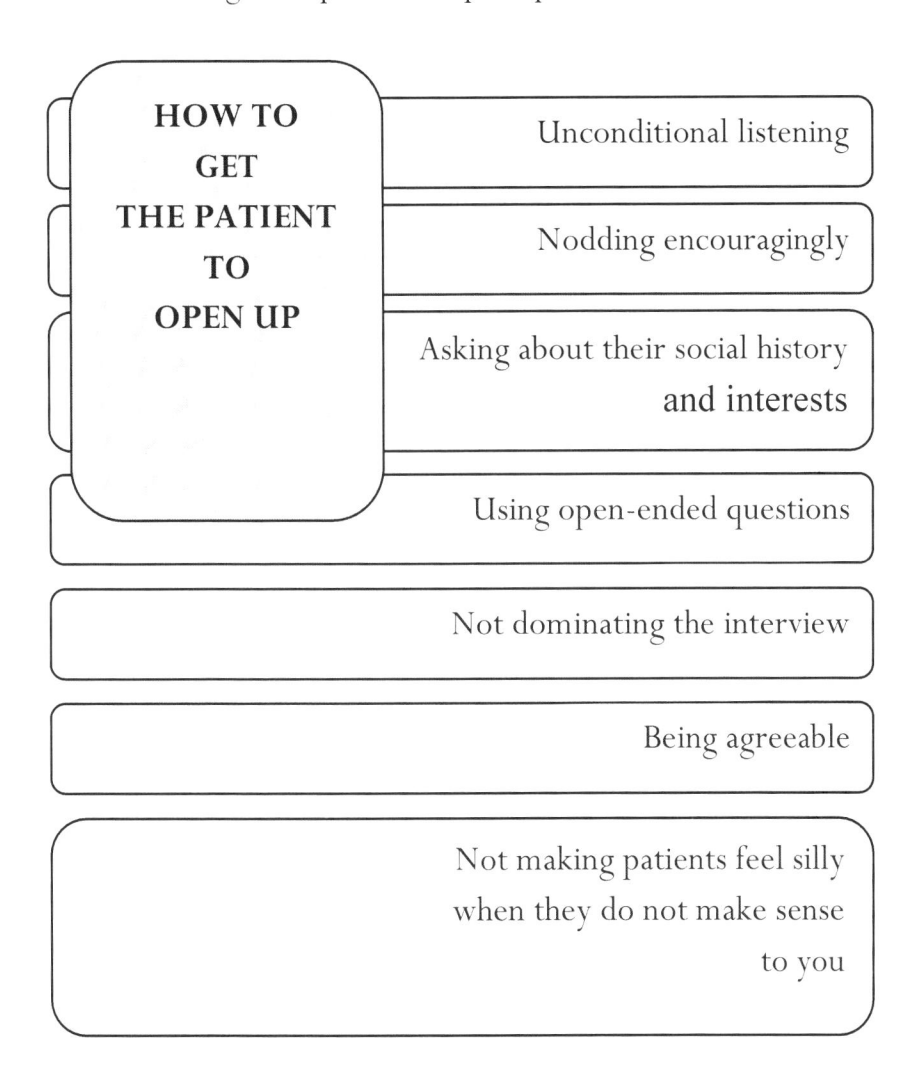

HOW TO GET THE PATIENT TO OPEN UP	
	Unconditional listening
	Nodding encouragingly
	Asking about their social history and interests
	Using open-ended questions
	Not dominating the interview
	Being agreeable
	Not making patients feel silly when they do not make sense to you

ESTABLISHING AN EMOTIONAL CONNECTION

We have established that good people skills give you an edge in this profession. Being caring, respectful, patient and warm will take you far and lay the groundwork for a successful dentist-patient relationship. You must realize that in this day and age, it is insufficient for a patient to be satisfied with your actual dentistry; you must also establish an emotional connection if you want the patient to remain a long-time customer. Establishing an emotional connection takes time; one appointment is insufficient. Nevertheless, you can lay the foundation for a long-term relationship during the first appointment. Accept the relationship as long term, and your communication will automatically adjust. You are sure to find some common ground eventually, and this is when a connection will form.

Table 4: Creating an emotional connection.

CREATING AN EMOTIONAL CONNECTION

- Respect your patient
- Value your patient's time
- Practice active and attentive listening
- Be curious and interested
- Express empathy
- Be kind
- Share something personal about yourself

AVOIDING A SOLICITOR'S APPROACH—SEPARATING HEALTHCARE AND BUSINESS

I once had a meeting with a solicitor when buying a property. As I was speaking, he was openly timing me, which made him look insincere and untrustworthy. I never went back to him again, so he lost me as a client. I am certain that he practiced this approach regularly, which means that he probably ended up losing many other clients. Business without a personal touch may be effective in the short term, but your patients will never recommend you or trust you if you take a "solicitor's approach". It is essential for relationship building to precede financial gain. I once had a patient who could not tolerate dental examinations. She had to drink water every 5 minutes because she was very anxious. I spent hours with her building trust (for which I was not paid). Two years later, she is having extensive restorative work without any problems and has referred two patients to me. She trusts that I am looking after her best interests before my financial gain.

I am not implying that financial gain is unimportant. What I am trying to say is that it is essential to remember that you are a healthcare professional and that it is perfectly normal for some patients to need more time than others.

Five

Presentation of a Treatment Plan

A successful presentation of a treatment plan involves delivering solutions in a manner that is appropriate for the patient.

Table 5: Objectives for a successful treatment presentation.

OBJECTIVES FOR A SUCCESSFUL TREATMENT PRESENTATION
The patient • feels at ease and not prejudiced; • has discussed treatment aspects freely; • feels that all of his or her questions have been answered; • has had the opportunity to openly reflect on his or her dental health; • has a brief understanding of your proposed plan; • leaves the surgery in a state of emotional stability; • feels as though he or she has been involved in decision making and planning; • feels comfortable to return with questions.

You probably can note that most of the objectives presented above are not measurable. The only important factor is how you make your patients feel and what you make them think.

PREPARE

Stefan and I once had a meeting with an interior designer because I wanted to purchase custom wardrobes and furniture for our new flat. The designer took measurements and asked us for one week to prepare a 3D plan. We knew that it would be expensive, but we also really wanted what he had to offer. One week later, we met the designer at the showroom at the appointed time. He was late because he was talking to another customer; moreover, he had not had time to prepare the promised 3D plan. Instead, he gave us a couple of catalogues to go through that showed different types of furniture. He described tables as round or square. It was a mess—the poorest presentation that I have ever heard! We were interested in purchasing furniture worth thousands of pounds, and the designer had not even bothered to pick out furniture that would suit our requests. Moreover, he wasted 1.5 hours of our time going back and forth in catalogues. My first thought was, "*If this is how unprofessional he is before we have paid for his services, imagine then how unprofessional he will be after!*" His disorganized attitude also made me question the quality of the custom-made furniture. Obviously, we did not buy anything from him.

The benefits of rehearsing your treatment-plan presentations are endless. You will feel more confident and calm. You will be more prepared for questions, and the rehearsal will make you anticipate and think about the questions that you could be asked. Make sure you know every detail of your proposed treatment so that you are prepared to answer any questions without hesitation. The outcomes of the presentation are directly related to the work that you put into it. Patients are more likely to commence treatment if they understand you, see that you know what you are talking about and feel that you have made an effort.

SETTING THE SCENE

When Stefan proposed, he took me to a historic place called Mdina in Malta. It was New Year's Eve, and I had my hair done and was wearing a new dress. We went to a Michelin-starred restaurant and had an amazing dinner surrounded by lovely, happy people. Stefan proposed to me after dinner at a viewpoint outside the restaurant. It is a sweet memory. Now, imagine if Stefan took me to the same viewpoint in Mdina on a mid-week afternoon and casually popped the question. Even worse, imagine if he just gave me the ring after discussing the practicalities of marriage. My memory would be totally different. Stefan made an effort to set the scene for his proposal, and it obviously had the results that he wanted. The same principles apply for presenting a treatment plan to a patient.

Setting the scene for a treatment presentation means wearing professional attire and looking like what you are selling. It also means paying attention to every little detail such as which music you are playing, how tidy your workspace is, and how you position your chair in relation to your patient's chair. Efforts should be made for the patient to be able to see, experience and feel what the planned treatment is about. Marcus Hines, author of *"Dental Implant Marketing"*, very cleverly related buying expensive dental treatment to buying a car. You obviously want to sit in a car, test drive it and experience it before you buy. The same principles apply to dental treatment; patients want to experience, see and feel what they are buying.

I usually set up two chairs, one for me and one for the patient, in front of my computer. Sitting next to each other removes barriers. It also communicates agreement and friendliness. A printed copy of the treatment plan is in front of us. Radiographs are shown on the computer screen. I have a second computer with the patient's photographs. On the table I have placed models that relate to the treatment and a mirror so that the patient can see which tooth I am referencing. All of this makes it look like I have made an effort for the patient to be able to follow what I am saying. Patients are not stupid. If they understand you and trust you, they will agree with you. I can tell you that this not only gets the patient excited about their treatment but also protects you from dental malpractice complaints because you have made every possible effort to explain your plan.

KNOW YOUR PATIENT
Your treatment plan delivery should be tailored to your patient's personality, communication style, needs and goals. The only way to learn this information is by spending sufficient time with and listening to your patients talk about themselves. Do not make assumptions about your patients and their intelligence or what you think they would want to know. Spending time creating common ground will also reveal emotional triggers that you can incorporate into your treatment presentation.

ATTRACTING YOUR PATIENT'S ATTENTION
The best-selling author and communication expert, Nancy Duarte states that the secret to an idea's success is how it is communicated. Patients' attention will wander if you are boring, unclear, and lack confidence. They are more likely to listen to your idea if there is something in it for them, if what you say is valuable, if you are positive and if you communicate that you believe in it yourself.

DELIVERY OF INFORMATION

AVOID LECTURING
Avoid focusing your presentations on yourself and what you can provide. Despite your best intentions, your patients will never thank you for lecturing and showing off. Lecturing will insult their intelligence or, at best, make them feel dumb. Negative wording such as "no", "but"

and "however" may portray you as trying to look superior. Instead, focus your presentation on what the patient can have, and use positive wording.

STORYTELLING
This concept can be highly effective and it involves engaging the patient by telling a story or using a familiar analogy. Make the story realistic, personal and relevant. Imagine how much better you can communicate your point when you tell the story of your grandfather's dentures, which were progressively loosening, and how, to his embarrassment, they fell out as he was enjoying a nice piece of steak at a fancy restaurant—as opposed to saying, "Implants will support your dentures".

A TAILORED APPROACH
Consider your patients' preferred learning styles and need for information. Some patients prefer information in writing, and some are more interactive. Let patients know beforehand that you have prepared information in writing because this will reduce the pressure that they experience; they won't feel like they have to memorize everything you say. They also won't feel rushed into making a decision on the spot.

THINK ELEVATOR PITCH
A presentation is a pitch, and the patient is a customer who has the ability to accept or decline your proposal. Some dentists shy away from this fact. They do not realize that most patients love being sold to! They love it because it makes them feel like valued customers who are in control of their treatments. An elevator pitch involves making an enduring impression in a short time frame. What would you say if you only had 60 seconds? Thinking about this in detail will encourage you

to focus on the main points without overwhelming your patient. Keep in mind that patients will not recall most of what you say; it is therefore useful to focus on the most important aspects of their treatment. The fine details should be covered in a written treatment plan.

WHAT IS THE MOST CONFUSING ASPECT?

Something that is very straightforward to you may be completely confusing to your patient. Think about the aspect of your treatment plan that will cause the most confusion and detail it in writing. Slow your speech and emphasize key words by pausing while ensuring that your patient is engaging at each pause. Always ask if the patient is following by saying, *"Am I making sense to you?"* or *"Am I explaining this well?"* This prevents the patient from feeling confused; you are highlighting that the reason that they do not understand you is your inability to deliver the information in an appropriate manner. Do not use dental jargon, which may come across as unsympathetic or as though you are attempting to mislead your patient.

LANGUAGE AND SLANG

Although frequent use of slang may suggest that your dialogue is too informal and unfit for the dental surgery context, some patients prefer an informal setting. It is best to be your genuine self and attempt to adjust your language to your patient by modelling the type of language that the patient uses.

READING YOUR PATIENT

Accurately interpreting your patient's communication will enable you to further tailor your approach during the presentation. A patient who is ready for the next appointment will look you in the eyes and smile or laugh (if you are funny). You might also find that a patient will mimic your non-verbal language when he or she agrees with you. A patient who is unready for treatment or who disagrees with you will raise his or her eyebrows, frown, or narrow the eyes. The patient might also tilt his or her head to the side and purse their lips. The body language will be tense, and there will be uncomfortable pauses in the discussion.

BLACK AND WHITE

Imagine a stand with 10 types of decadent desserts, some more expensive than others. They all have their advantages and disadvantages; some are decorated with local produce, whereas others are decorated with exotic, previously frozen fruits from Africa. All of the desserts are supposed to taste amazing, but you have no idea what will suit your palate because you are not a pastry chef and you have not experienced any of the flavours before. For that reason, you will choose one of the decadent desserts and hope that you will enjoy it, but you will always feel that you might have missed out on something better. The experience could even take away the pleasure of having your chosen dessert while you watch other customers buying what you did not choose.

In the same manner, presenting several good treatment options to patients will only create confusion and, at worst, paralysis. This approach could also frighten patients because they might feel that they may be missing out by choosing the wrong option. This could delay a patient's decision, resulting in a decision not to obtain treatment at all. Worse yet, the patient could choose a treatment only to find that he or she is not satisfied with the choice. Your presentation of treatment options must take into account that our brains do not like information presented in "grey". Do not complicate the information. Instead, deliver it in "black and white". Your patient should be able to easily understand and distinguish between the options, and the advantages and disadvantages should be clearly defined. Just as a pastry chef would make me feel better by telling me *"great choice!"*, your opinion and feedback related to your patients' choices matter and will make them feel at ease about their decisions.

CHUNKING

A complex case will require a long treatment plan with many options. Simplify the delivery of your information by grouping the information together into categories. This approach makes it less confusing for your patient to make an informed decision. Studies show that memory retention is improved when information is presented in categories.

CONCLUDING YOUR PRESENTATION

The end is as important as the beginning. This is your last opportunity to make a positive and lasting impression on your patient. Practice the following strategies to ensure that you make the most of this opportunity.

1. Patients generally forget 60% of what you tell them. Encourage your patients to ask questions and invite them into the discussion. This will increase the likelihood that your patients will remember your conversations. Very few patients will have no questions. If they have no questions, it is probably because you have confused them or not encouraged them.
2. Summarize the main points as in your elevator pitch.
3. Emphasize the benefits.
4. Ask for feedback. Asking, *"How does this sound?"* is a good way to obtain immediate feedback on your treatment plan.
5. Advise your patients about how to make follow-up appointments and refer to your receptionist using his/her first name. Reassure patients that the receptionist has been informed and will take good care of them.

6. Encourage (do not force) patients to make their first appointment and thank them for their time.

RESPONDING TO "THANK YOU"

"Thank you" is a positive and sincere expression that should be met with an equally positive and sincere reply. Your choice of words matters, and your response should be adjusted to your environment. Responding with *"sure"* or *"don't mention it"* can seem too casual and inappropriate for the setting. *"No problem"* is another inappropriate expression because the patient may wonder why it would ever be a problem. Moreover, you are using two negative words together ("No" and "Problem").

Diane Gottsman, an etiquette expert, recommends three vital components when responding to a *"Thank you"*:

- **Sincerity**: Patients will feel heard and respected.
- **Warmth**: A mild smile and eye contact will enhance your words.
- **Tone:** Do not mumble. A smile will also result in a happier-sounding voice.

YOU ONLY HAVE ONE CHANCE!

You will not retain your patients' trust once that trust has been lost. You do not get a do-over. Make sure that you have pulled out all the stops the first time around.

Table 6: Summary of key aspects of a successful presentation.

KEY ASPECTS FOR A SUCCESSFUL TREATMENT PRESENTATION
• Do not judge • Do not assume • Do not blame • Be personal • Involve your patient • Do not worry about fees; people buy you and you are awesome! • Speak confidently and be clear. Patients do want your opinion and you do know what is best • Use positive and affirmative language • Communicate benefits • Make suggestions, not decisions • Do not worry about rejections; they are not personal • Remember, what you say before treatment is an explanation, and what you say after is an excuse

Six

Influencing Patients

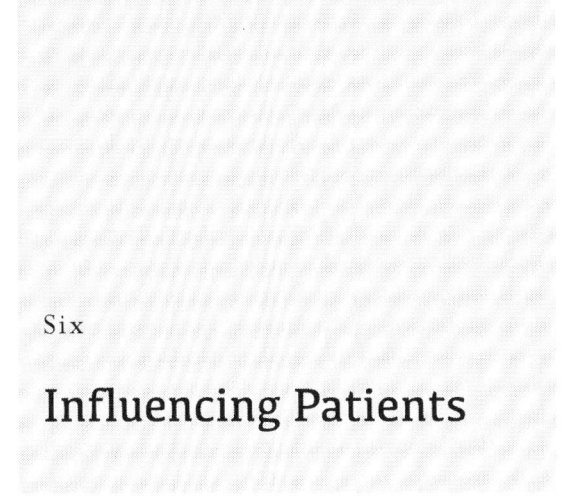

Patients are creatures of emotion. You will have to change how they feel if you are going to be able to change how they think. Do not assume that a patient is ignorant because he or she declines treatment. Probe deeper by asking, *"May I ask why...?"* and *"How would you like me to help you?"* Patients tend to decline treatment when they fail to understand their benefits of treatment. Ensuring that you communicate the correct benefits will result in increased treatment acceptance.

STRATEGIES FOR INFLUENCING PATIENTS

1. Be empathetic.
2. Communicate benefits and show the patient how those benefits can be reaped.
3. Emphasize the goal. Tell the patient to visualize how they will look and feel once treatment is finished. For example, when suggesting 3 monthly hygiene visits, I always mention that the patient will no longer need to attend frequent hygiene appointments once we achieve a perfect plaque score. Talk about the future rather than the present.

4. Involve your patients and give them full control; they are more likely to follow through with treatment if they believe that it is their idea. They will also cope better with treatment that they have chosen.
5. Use worst-case scenarios (note that this approach does not work on everyone; you must know your patients to ensure that you are not scaring them away). For example, I have some fabulous models of resorbed mandibles, and I simply say, *"This is what happens when we lose teeth"* while showing them the resorption patterns.
6. Do not reject a "No". It is not personal, and it is not an insult. Respond instead as follows: *"I am just here to advise you. They are your teeth, and you decide what you want to have done. I leave this up to you because you know what is best for your teeth"*.
7. Be easy-going. Do not set a deadline; no one is going to die. Tell your patients that the sooner the treatment is done the better, but that they should not feel stressed about it. Nine out of ten times, this will result in treatment acceptance within a month.
8. Do not take anger, frustration or irritation to heart. You are just a messenger stating your observations. Patients do not know you, and they are not aiming to hurt you when you deliver news that they do not want to hear.
9. Be a happy dentist. Smile a bit and do everything you can to promote a friendly environment. No one wants to work with or be around a grumpy person, let alone a grumpy dentist.
10. Make it easy for patients to make subsequent appointments and ask them about their appointment preferences. This shows that you are interested in accommodating them. Explain what the next appointment is for and how long it will take.

MOTIVATIONAL INTERVIEWING

Preaching or lecturing to a patient will be met with irritation and resistance to change. Motivational interviewing is a patient-centred approach that recognizes the internal factors that are resistant to change. Sobell and Sobell (2008) have written a very helpful review that advises the following strategies:

1. Ask for permission to talk about the problem.
2. Use non-confrontational language.
3. Offer to help and be supportive.
4. Be empathetic.
5. Observe your patient's non-verbal and verbal language. Is the patient tense or interested? Is the patient confident that he or she can change?
6. Ask open-ended questions to promote a discussion.
7. Listen attentively! What do the patient's words mean? Is the patient ready for a change?
8. Normalize the patient's behaviour. Telling the patient that the situation is common and completely normal or that you have seen worse will make them feel less embarrassed.

Seven

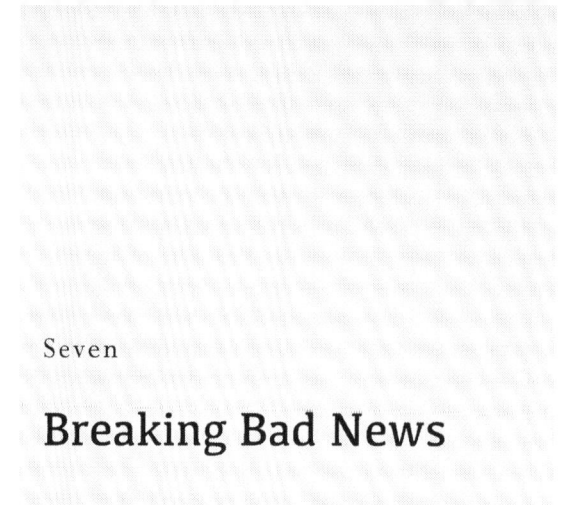

Breaking Bad News

I once treated a 70-year-old man who presented with an extensive infection around an upper molar tooth. I showed him the radiograph and explained that it would be best to extract the tooth. I did not think twice about delivering this news because I thought that in light of the fact that some of his other teeth were missing, he would not care very much. When I turned to look at him, his eyes were wet. I felt terrible! I had judged a book by its cover! For the average patient, losing teeth is a traumatic, devastating and life-changing experience. It results in terrible insecurity that one may be perceived as old or in poor health.

The definition of "bad news" varies from patient to patient. For one patient it may mean that they need a simple filling, and to another it may mean that they require multiple extractions. The initial consultation and assessment visits are your only opportunities to avoid judging the book (the patient) by its cover. This is when you will have the ability to learn what bad news means to your patient and to tailor your delivery accordingly. The delivery of bad news will always remain an unpleasant but essential part of dentistry, and if not thought through, it can be met with surprise or shock.

Your method of delivering bad news has the potential to either make or break your relationship with patients because it can affect their expectations and attitudes. It might also influence their satisfaction with both you and your treatment. The patient's perception of and reaction to bad news will depend on his or her life experiences, personality, culture, social milieu and mental hardiness.

Table 7: Key principles of delivering bad news.

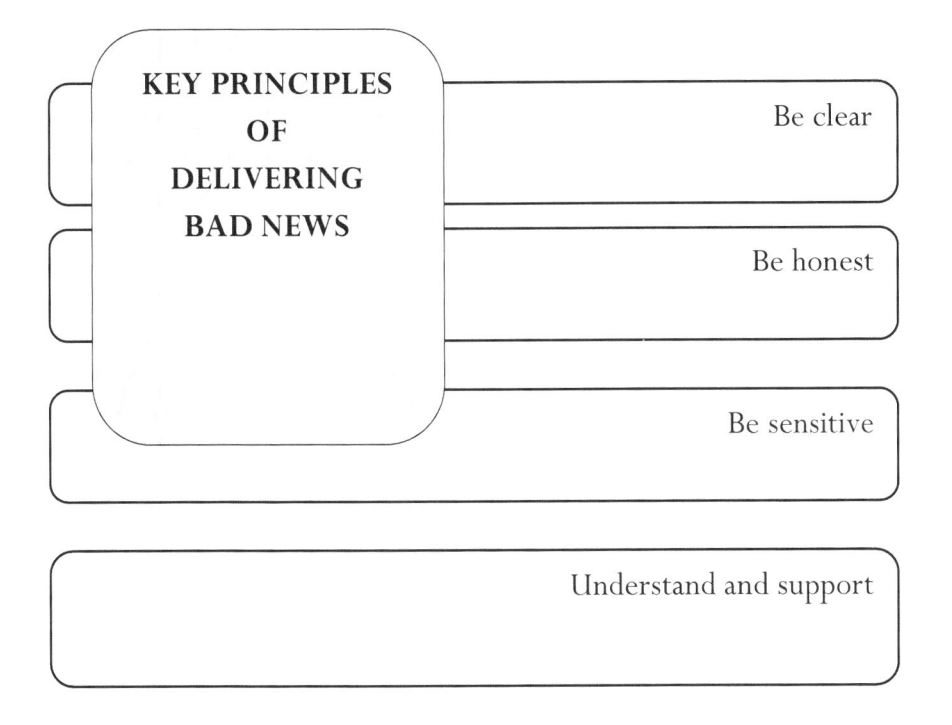

KEY PRINCIPLES OF DELIVERING BAD NEWS
Be clear
Be honest
Be sensitive
Understand and support

SETTING

The setting should communicate privacy, friendliness and safety. The environment should be perceived as confidential; to avoid interruptions, the door should not be open. The ideal setting is away from the dental chair, which is an emotionally charged environment in any event. The patient should feel comfortable to express his or her emotions as a reaction to the bad news.

THE HUMAN ELEMENT
As you now know, non-verbal communication adds meaning to your words and is an essential element in preventing misunderstandings. Therefore, you cannot deliver bad news in writing or on the phone because you would lose the ability to read your patient and gauge his or her emotional state in relation to the news. Moreover, you lose the ability to control the state in which your patient receives the news. You are not helping yourself if you catch the patient at a bad time.

PUT YOURSELF IN YOUR PATIENT'S SHOES
How would you want bad news to be delivered to yourself or your family members? Think about that and you will instantly feel more empathy for the patient. Realize that the patient is not a dentist, and use language that the patient understands and to which he or she can relate.

LAY THE GROUNDWORK TO READY THE PATIENT
How well does the patient understand his or her condition? To avoid surprise, take time to explain the patient's current dental status. Use "warning statements" to prepare the patient emotionally, and watch the patient's reaction after each statement. Continue prepping until the patient seems ready to hear more. You could say, *"Some teeth are not so healthy"* or *"Some teeth are doing more harm than good"*. Ensure that the patient is receptive to the final delivery. Wait for an invitation, which might be in the form of a question. Simply asking, *"Shall we discuss your X-rays today?"* or *"Shall we go into detail about your tooth today?"* is a good way of assessing readiness.

REASONS BEFORE FEELINGS
Always talk logic and facts before bad news. The patient will be too emotional to comprehend and remember details once the bad news has been delivered.

DO NOT OVERLOAD
Focus on the bad news only and do not go into detail. Work with emotions at this stage, and reassure the patient that a written letter will be provided to document the conversation. Patients will not have the capacity to make decisions once they have received bad news. For that reason, it is important not to present any estimates or force patients to immediately schedule a treatment appointment. Offer the patient a free follow-up appointment to discuss the treatment plan.

EXPLAIN
Suggest treatment options and the consequences of not receiving your recommended treatment. Patients want what is best for them. If you use the correct wording, they will also choose the correct treatment. For example, my mentor, Jonathon, would say, *"The infection is eating up your jaw bone"* instead of talking about the physiology of bone resorption.

POSITIVE WORDING AND POSITIVE OUTLOOK
Always introduce bad news with good news. Patients will understand what you are getting at by your non-verbal language either way. Using negative wording will make your bad news sound worse. Avoid negatively charged expressions such as *"Unfortunately"* or *"I have bad news"*. Emphasize the end result; show photos and models so that the patient can focus on the end result instead of the current situation. Talk about a similar patient who has had the same treatment. Even better, show photos of the treatment results for that patient.

SILENCE AND PAUSING
Respect that patients might need time to process the news. Give them the time that they need and provide emotional support. Silence enables patients to process information and explore their emotional responses to the news. Wait for a cue from the patient before you continue.

PROVIDE GUIDANCE
Advise the patient on the next step and encourage follow-through. You have to do this for patients because they will be too consumed with other thought processes to follow through with practicalities.

HONESTY
Most patients appreciate an honest approach if it is handled with sensitivity. Usually, honesty is better than trying to overlook or ignore the problem. The sooner you can introduce the bad news, the better—for them and for you. Delaying the inevitable will not make it easier for either of you.

YOU ARE THE MESSENGER
It is not personal, and it is not your fault that the patient is being given bad news. You are the messenger, and the patient will see you as just that if you deliver the news appropriately. Hiding bad news is not the way to gain a patient's trust. Accept that patients may cope by being defensive and in denial. Confrontations will only further increase their anxiety. At the end of treatment, most patients will be grateful for having been informed of their situation.

PRACTICE AND PREPARE
Practice your delivery of bad news if you are unsure about which method to use or how you sound. This will make you more confident, and you will have subconsciously thought about possible questions that you may be asked.

Eight

Communicating Fees

In dental school, we are taught a set of highly specialized skills, but only a few of us have been taught how to successfully sell that particular skill set. People who run sales courses are not usually dental professionals and thus will never be able to completely relate to us. For example, you cannot demand that a patient signs a treatment plan without having had a chance to consider it. You must remain ethical and remember that you are a health care professional and that the patient's best interest comes before financial gain. Nevertheless, we cannot practice our skills if we cannot sell them: it is as simple as that!

MONEY

Money is a dirty little thing that people do not talk about; however, they think about it most of the time. It is a private matter that can make people feel insecure, frustrated and angry. Talking about money is talking about class, and who wants to say that they do not belong to a high class? Saying that you have plenty of money can be frowned upon as bragging, whereas saying that you have too little could make you look irresponsible or uneducated. For most people, money is also security; patients will not part with security unless they trust you and your promise of a valuable return. For this reason, it is a bad idea to talk about high fees before you and your patient have formed a relationship and you are trusted to be able to deliver what the patient wants and needs.

Figure 2: The meaning of money.

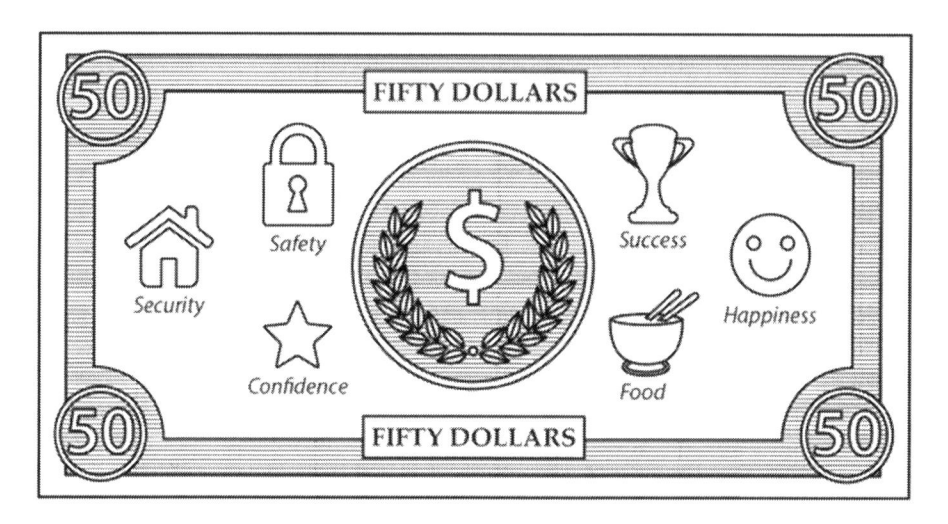

WHY IT IS DIFFICULT TO TALK ABOUT MONEY

I wasn't always good at talking about money; this is a skill that I have picked up over the years. It can be extremely difficult to name your price—what YOU and YOUR services are worth. Talking about money is also directly related to confidence and believing in what you are selling. A money discussion will be no problem at all if you believe in your fees and that you and your services are worthy of them.

Table 8: Why it is difficult to talk about money.

WHY IT IS DIFFICULT TO TALK ABOUT MONEY
• You do not believe in your fees • You do not believe you are worthy of your fees • You are afraid of rejection and objections • You feel that you are rejected and not valued when your prices are rejected • You are very risk averse • You are generally uncomfortable talking about money

As you can see, it isn't as simple as saying, "*I just don't like to talk about money*". There is usually a deeper reason, which you will need to identify. Your perception of and relationship with money will influence how people around you (including patients) view money. For example, I was always taught to not talk about money as a child. For that reason, I found it incredibly difficult to name my price when I started to work as a dentist. I associated asking for money as being greedy. Many times, I felt like I was asking for too much. Are you allowing your judgements and confidence to get in the way of offering treatments that could benefit your patients?

HOW DO YOU FEEL WHEN YOU LET GO OF YOUR HARD-EARNED MONEY?

I have encountered some terrible sales people. Some are foolish enough to judge me by what I wear, and some are ignorant enough to make decisions for me based on what they think they know about me. Good salespeople will not ask where I work or what I do unless it is relevant to my product choice, and they will not make judgements based on what I am wearing. Customers buy when they feel that their hard-earned money is used on something that is equal to the hours of work and effort that has been put into earning that money. However, the fact remains that patients will never be happy to see their money depart, regardless of how wealthy they are. Thinking about your own feelings and behaviours when buying will help you understand what your patient is going through when given a proposal that equates to a month's work or more. It is not as simple as communicating benefits and value; it is about communicating long-term benefits and value. It is also about communicating not only long-term happy feelings but also the guarantee of a valuable return. The most important factor, however, is to show that you appreciate the value of the money that you are requesting. Patients will trust you with their money if you value it as much as they do.

WHAT IS THE VALUE OF GOOD DENTAL TREATMENT?

Dental treatment is one of the most difficult products to sell: it is invisible, and patients cannot appreciate it until it has been delivered to them. A few months ago, I needed a composite filling to restore a lower molar tooth, for which I was charged £300. Three hundred pounds is a very fair price for the excellent service that I received. To my embarrassment, however, I found that a £300 handbag would have made me happier. It was my common sense that prioritized dental care. The £300 did give me a functional tooth, but not the joy and excitement that a designer handbag would have given me. This realization was ground breaking and gave me great insight into the challenge of selling dental treatment. It made me realize that dental treatment must be sold in terms of its benefits, just like a designer handbag or a car.

Very few people will see value in dentistry if it is not communicated to them. They may accept treatment for the same reasons that I accepted treatment. Like me, however, they are likely to feel the sting of asking, *"What did I just pay for?"* Costs are rarely an issue if they are appropriately justified and presented to the patient. Patients will buy what they perceive is good value and what makes them happy. Ranting about titanium and ceramics is not going to make patients happy! Instead, talking about youthfulness and having the ability to eat an apple will.

"YOUR FEES ARE HIGH"

Most dentists have been faced with this statement at least once. The best way to deal with this statement is to grab it by its horns and just go for it! Accept that for the average person, dentistry is expensive; then again, so are designer shoes, and I still buy those! People shy away from the word "expensive" because it is often seen as a synonym for "overpriced". You are more likely to feel comfortable with the word "expensive" if you interpret it as a word that denotes high-end, top-quality dentistry.

It is expensive to have a mouth full of implants; the lab bills are expensive, and there is a great deal of work involved. Agreeing with your patients when they are shocked by your estimate is the first step to gaining patients' acceptance. This is an approach that I learned from my mentor, Jonathon, who simply responds by saying, *"Yes, it is expensive"*. Being in agreement will show that you are eager to begin a relationship with the patient and that you are on their side. No one wants to get closer to a person with whom they disagree.

YES, YES, YES!

We have a deep-rooted need to be happy when we buy. This is why, for example, touristy hotspots are flooded with people selling overpriced and poor-quality knick-knacks with little long-term value or use to buyers. We are happy and relaxed when on holiday, and we like to spend this happy time parting with our hard-earned money. We also like to buy so that we can later remind ourselves of those happy times. In the same way, your patient is more likely to agree to treatment if he or she is happy, relaxed and agreeable. Patients will not agree to treatment if they are stressed, rushed or worried, nor will they agree to treatment if they do not agree with you. The first step in selling is therefore to make patients happy and relaxed (you have to know your patients to be able to do this). The second step is to ask a few leading questions. You must be confident that your patient will answer *"yes"* to all of your questions (again, you have to know your patient to be able to do this). The final question is simply, *"Would you like to proceed with the treatment?"*

THE BIG 5 FOR COMMUNICATING FEES

1. EMOTIONAL HOT BUTTONS

This concept is common within the field of marketing. It is essentially based upon what makes people buy what we sell. The hot buttons must be communicated as you sell your dentistry.

Table 9: Dental treatment hot buttons.

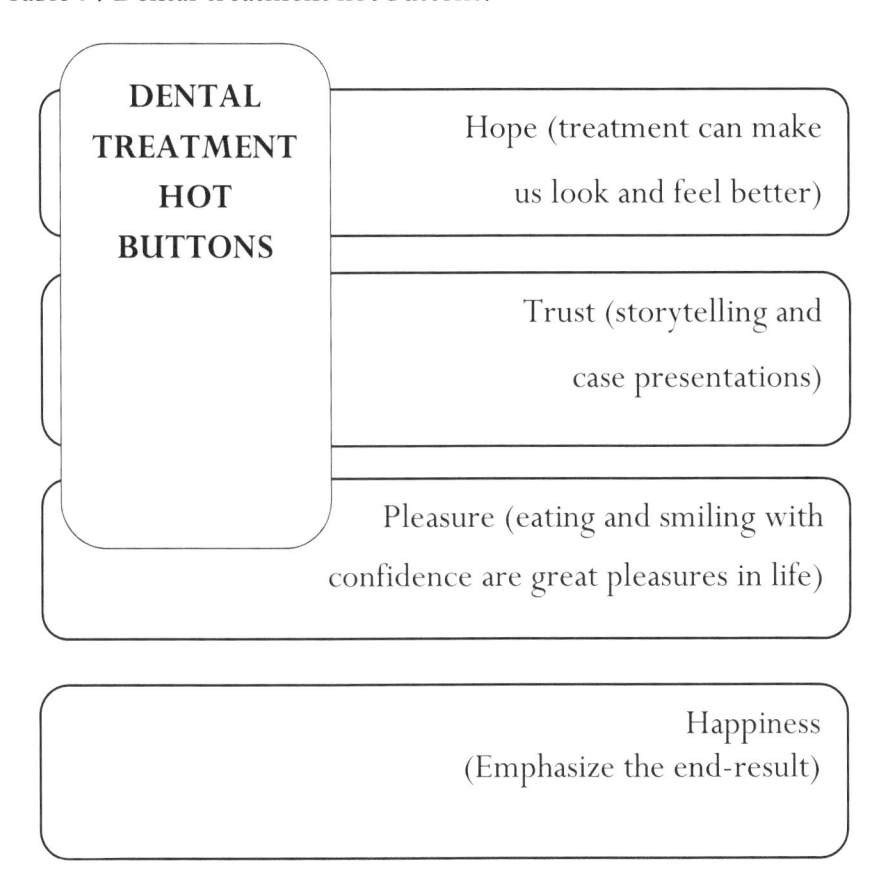

DENTAL TREATMENT HOT BUTTONS
- Hope (treatment can make us look and feel better)
- Trust (storytelling and case presentations)
- Pleasure (eating and smiling with confidence are great pleasures in life)
- Happiness (Emphasize the end-result)

2. CONFIDENCE

Believe in your proposed treatment and what you are charging. This belief will resonate with your patients. Why should a patient believe in your fees if you don't believe in them yourself?

3. DO NOT CONVINCE AND AVOID DESPERATION

We all have bills to pay, but this should not be the reason to sell dental treatment. Showing the patient that you are simply interested in their benefits and happiness will communicate that their decision is not personal. They are more likely to agree to treatment if the pressure is off and you have a laid-back attitude.

4. HONESTY AND INTEGRITY
You must believe in your prices and that both you and your treatment are worthy of them. Honesty and integrity resonate through your non-verbal communication. Patients will sense your good intentions and honesty. In the same way, they will be able to sense if you are selling treatment for your own benefit.

5. SAY GOOD-BYE TO JUDGEMENTS
You have absolutely no idea which patients will agree to treatment. Remember that failing to inform your patients of their treatment options is neglectful.

Table 10: Dos of communicating fees.

DOS OF COMMUNICATING FEES
Before • Prepare your patient. Surprising the patient can result in a defensive reaction. • Prepare yourself; it is unprofessional to not know your own fees. **During** • Communicate confidence and empathy. • Relaxed body language is essential. You want the fees to sound good and to have a feel-good factor surrounding the conversation. • Be clear. There is nothing worse than a person who says, "This will be around £300". It looks unorganized and communicates poor confidence in your fees. • Be genuine, transparent, enthusiastic and passionate. **After** • Await the reaction. Imagine a build-up with a BANG at the end. • Be open-minded and cooperative. • Be flexible, but stick to what you believe in. It shows great character and confidence. • Listen attentively to show that you care.

Table 11: Don'ts of communicating fees.

DON'TS OF COMMUNICATING FEES
• Reducing fees communicates that you do not believe in them and that they are set too high. • Excusing fees communicates that you are not worthy of what you charge. • Being emotional will confuse and derail you. • Convincing shows desperation and makes it look like the treatment is all about you, not the patient. • Arguing or disagreeing communicates disrespect, and patients will not trust you with their money. No one wants to hear that they are wrong. • Do not give a naked number; associate the number with value.

REJECTION

To some extent, we all have a fear of rejection. People who worry uncontrollably about rejection tend to practice defensive, unempathetic behaviour. It is vital to recognize that rejections are not necessarily personal. Patients may be caught off-guard when you disclose your estimate. Some patients are just naturally defensive or cautious, and you may find that they belong to one of the following groups:

1. They like a bargain and enjoy the experience of negotiating the price.
2. They feel dumbfounded because they have not thought the treatment through.
3. They feel that they are being tricked because your competitor is offering the same treatment (of an inferior quality, of course) for half the price.

The solution is to find the reason for the rejection and change your approach accordingly. The solution is also to work on yourself to avoid becoming self-absorbed when a patient says *"No"*.

MOST IMPORTANTLY....

Do not forget that this is meant to be fun. It is meant to be an enjoyable experience for both you and the patient. Do not take things too seriously. Laugh and joke with your patients to create a connection. Relationship building is the essence of any business relationship. Patients who understand and trust you will believe in you and pay your fees. Remember that it is not what you are quoting but how you are quoting it.

Nine

Cross-Cultural Communication

Both culture and background—yours and your patients'—will influence your interpersonal communication (see the communication loop in Figure 1). Friendly behaviour in one culture could, for example, come across as strange and inappropriate in another. Knowledge of cultural differences can help us understand both ourselves and people who are different from us. Applying your knowledge on culture-specific differences will help you be more respectful and empathetic towards your patients who belong to cultures other than your own. Being able to tailor your communication to your patient will not only prevent misunderstandings but will also help to build the relationship. The recommendations in this chapter are generalizations and should not be considered universal.

EMOTIONAL VERSUS CONFRONTATIONAL

Erin Meyer, author of the "culture map", describes four divisions of cultures that influence how people tend to communicate and negotiate. Cultures can be categorized by how confrontational and emotionally expressive they are.

Table 12: Culture-specific emotional expressiveness by Erin Meyer.

Emotionally expressive / Confrontational
Israel, Russia, France, Spain

Emotionally expressive / Avoids confrontation
Brazil, India, Mexico, Saudi Arabia, Philippines

Emotionally inexpressive / Confrontational
Netherlands, Germany, Denmark

Emotionally inexpressive / Avoids confrontation
UK, Sweden, Korea, Japan

COMMUNICATION STYLES

VERBAL

Dupraw and Axner, authors of *"Working on common cross cultural communication challenges"*, write that Americans interpret a loud discussion as a fight or a reason to be alarmed. Conversely, Africans and Mediterranean perceive an increase in volume as a sign of an exciting conversation amongst friends and therefore see increased volume as completely normal. Meyer describes a raised voice, laughing, expressing emotions and making body contact as normal behaviour in regions such as South America and Saudi Arabia. The same behaviour in Scandinavia and the UK can be perceived as exaggerated, unprofessional or immature. The tactics that Meyer recommends include the following: adapting the way your disagreement is expressed to fit the other culture, learning how they build trust and avoiding yes/no questions, which can often cause cross-cultural clashes.

NON-VERBAL
Although facial expressions are universal, some cultures tend to emphasize them more than others. Mediterranean and Middle Eastern cultures use more dramatic facial expressions than Asian cultures do. It is essential for your facial expressions to remain neutral and represent the words you are speaking to avoid confusion. Patients from emotionally expressive cultures value the emotional connection and the process of getting to know one another before embarking on extensive treatment.

ATTITUDES TOWARDS CONFLICTS
According to Meyer, some cultures (e.g., France and Scandinavia) view expressing disagreement as a constructive discussion and a sign that you have processed the information. Other cultures (e.g., South America and Saudi Arabia) view disagreements as a sign of disrespect or something embarrassing that should be worked out quietly.

CONSENT
Patients from emotionally expressive cultures prefer an emotional connection before practical aspects such as consent forms or treatment plans are considered.

Contracts are also less common in countries in which the traditional legal system is less reliable. Presenting a consent form or treatment plan to sign to patients from these cultures could be perceived as a lack of trust or an attempt to trick them into a commitment. Therefore, ensure that you emphasize the reason for consent: it is to keep the patient informed.

DECISION MAKING

Your patients' decision-making abilities might be influenced by their culture—more specifically, decisions might be influenced by a patient's collectivist culture (e.g., the Middle East, Asia, South America) or individualistic culture (e.g., Scandinavia, Germany, UK, America). According to Dominik Guess, the author of "*Decision making in Individualistic and Collectivistic cultures*", individuals from individualistic cultures view themselves as relatively independent from others and are comfortable making their own decisions. In contrast, collectivist cultures stress the importance of relationships, roles and status within the social system. Therefore, decision making is collective, and both the family and the patient must be included in the treatment discussion.

APPOINTMENT ATTENDANCE

Attending appointments late is completely acceptable in some cultures and should not be mistaken as arrogance. You will need to account for this in your planning and inform the patient that attending on time is preferred, thus ensuring that the patient understands how you prefer to work.

AvGeri-Ann Galanti, the author of "*Caring for Patients from Different Cultures*", states that there are two types of time orientations: clock time and activity time. Someone who arrives at 3:15 for a 2:30 appointment is typically late; however, to someone who does not focus on clock time, both of these times represent the mid-afternoon. In countries with agriculture-based economies, people tend to be more relaxed about time; their pace is slower and more attuned to nature's rhythms. In contrast, industrialized nations avoid chaos by paying attention to clock time.

AVOIDING PITFALLS

Do not make the mistake of thinking that someone who looks like they are from a certain culture will possess traits specific to that culture. Furthermore, remember that your patients could be confused if your looks do not match your behaviour. I am a typical example of this phenomenon: I look Indian, but my mannerisms and values are Swedish. Sweden is the last place to which a person would relate my looks! What do you do if you are unsure about your patient's cultural background? You research your patient beforehand! As you have seen, being overly polite can actually offend.

Part III

The "Difficult" Patient

It is not possible to have 100% nice, friendly and polite patients. You cannot always control the state in which your patients come through your door. To some extent, however, you can control who becomes a long-term patient. If you want "good" patients, you have to learn to create them. The solution is not to run away or jump out of your window to avoid a difficult encounter. Instead, gather your confidence and face the music. Recognize that most often, the difficult patient has emerged because of problems in interpersonal communication and your failure to understand and empathize.

One

Self-Assessment

It is human nature and perfectly acceptable to be unable to see eye-to-eye with everyone. We naturally want to be around people with whom we identify and share values. However, you must recognize that you have a duty to care for your patients; therefore, it is in your interest to get along with them. Matthew Hussey, a relationship expert, suggests that to find your ideal partner, you should write down all the characteristics that you want from a partner. You should then aim to possess these characteristics yourself!

Most of the time, patients are a reflection of their dentists. You will find that patients who have been with you for a long time have a certain type of personality that is likely to be similar to yours. I have often encountered colleagues who complain about how difficult their patients are; some of the dramas I have heard of are quite astonishing. If you take a self-critical approach, nine out of ten times you will find a reason that the patient turned into a nightmare. More often than not, it is something that you have or have not said or done. Therefore, a little self-assessment is useful before you decide to blame the patient for being difficult.

BEING AGREEABLE

We often believe (and prefer) that other people think and act like us. Confident people do not feel the need to prove themselves right; instead, they appreciate different viewpoints, which enable them to understand different perspectives. A patient will not enjoy spending time with you if you do not respect his or her views. Patients want to feel good about themselves, which they will do if you listen to and respect their opinions and requests, even when you don't agree. Keep them happy by being agreeable.

VISUALIZE YOUR DREAM PATIENT AND YOUR NIGHTMARE PATIENT

You must know what you want from your patient list to understand your goals. Every dentist has a different "dream patient" and "nightmare patient". Visualize your dream patient and pay attention to the verbal and non-verbal language that you use with him or her. You will definitely find that your style of communication is significantly different when interacting with your "dream patient" than when interacting with your "nightmare patient". Apply your "good patient communication style" to your "nightmare patients" in the process of converting them to "dream patients". I have tried this myself, and it works!

TRAITS THAT COULD BRING OUT THE WORST IN PATIENTS

- Believing that you are always right.
- Insulting patients by telling them that they are wrong.
- Trying to convince patients to agree with you.

TRAITS THAT WILL BRING OUT THE BEST IN PATIENTS
- Being agreeable.
- Communicating that you are on the same side as your patients and that you are striving for the same goal.
- Communicating understanding and empathy by using the phrase, "*If I were you, I would feel just as you do*".
- Being diplomatic.
- Not treating a stranger; proceeding in baby steps until your patient is a friend and you are comfortable with each other.

FORGIVENESS AND PATIENCE
It is not always easy to be forgiving, especially when you feel like you have been wronged. A useful technique is to imagine your patient as a young child who does not know any better. This will instantly protect you from becoming upset or angry. Furthermore, realize that 99% of patients come from a place of good.

MAKE PEACE WITH COMPLAINTS
I was very nervous when I first realized that I had to have a complaints policy on my website. Although I used to see complaints as something awful, I have come to realize that complaints are gold. One verbal or written complaint will preserve your patient list because it will raise issues that are likely to be making many other patients unhappy. Therefore, do not punish a patient for complaining; instead, be grateful to him or her for providing you with a valuable opportunity to improve yourself and your services.

MANAGE YOUR OWN EXPECTATIONS

Avoid having unrealistic expectations. Patients will rarely act like us or say the things that we would say in a particular situation. You will be setting yourself up for disappointment and frustration if you expect your patients to be like you.

Two

The Human Element

DO NOT MAKE DENTISTRY A HABIT

At its worst, dentistry can be extremely stressful; there is time pressure, financial pressure, patient management, staff management and clinical aspects that all must be in focus. Sometimes dentistry feels like a rat race, and you may forget that the person in the chair is a living patient with a beating heart. Performing the same treatments day after day can also transform them into habits. A habit is the brain's ability to perform a task by transforming it to autopilot mode. This can explain, for example, why we sometimes find ourselves turning into the driveway after a familiar drive without having any recollection of how we got there.

Turning on to autopilot mode when practicing dentistry is unlikely to affect the quality of clinical treatment, but it will have an effect on how you connect with your patient because you will lose focus and miss important non-verbal cues. The patient is likely to sense the disconnect and your lack of mental presence, which could result in anxiety. Always remember that patients may forget what you say to them, but they will never forget how you have made them feel.

EMPATHY

Patients have two basic needs: the need for factual information and the need for emotional support and empathy. Empathy is what makes us human and what connects us to each other. Empathy is the ability to put yourself in someone else's shoes by showing that you care and are concerned for them. Communicating empathy is about acknowledging your patients' emotions without telling them that you know how they feel. This approach makes your patients feel valued, which will in turn build trust, aid in relationship building and normalize hostile situations. It is a skill that begins with practicing emotional management by controlling how you anticipate, permit and respond to your patients' emotional needs (Curtis and McConnell, 2012). Your patients will feel much more at ease around you when their emotions are validated without interruption or judgement.

Table 13: How to communicate empathy.

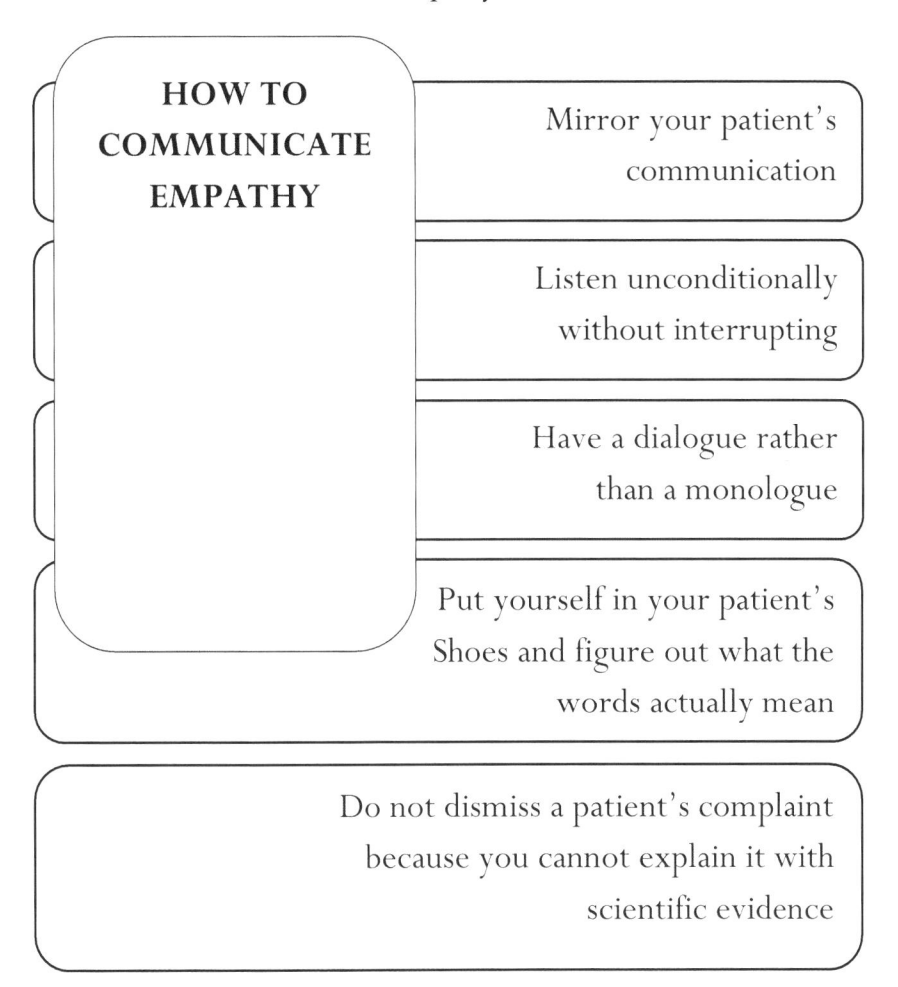

HOW TO COMMUNICATE EMPATHY
Mirror your patient's communication
Listen unconditionally without interrupting
Have a dialogue rather than a monologue
Put yourself in your patient's Shoes and figure out what the words actually mean
Do not dismiss a patient's complaint because you cannot explain it with scientific evidence

SYMPATHY

Being sympathetic is the ability to be able to feel sorry for someone by offering compassion. The key is to not speak for the patient, but instead to let him or her be. Your communication should reflect that you are there for your patients if they need you. Telling patients who are craving sympathy that you know how they feel will likely make them feel belittled and less important. The conversation should focus on your patient, not on you and your experiences.

VULNERABILITY AND TRUST

Being vulnerable involves exposing your emotions and yourself. It is something that we tend to do as we develop trust in another person. Showing vulnerability by letting your guard down will enable your patients to see you as the person you are instead of viewing you as a stereotypical dentist. It will make them recognize that you, too, have feelings and that your profession does not necessarily define who you are.

Being vulnerable signals to patients that you have trust in them. As a result, they are bound to return the favour by letting their guard down. Trust is the essence of a long-lasting relationship. You know that you have succeeded in establishing a long-lasting relationship when your patients decide to share highly personal facts, indicating that they trust you.

HONESTY

Be honest and always treat your patients the way you would want you or your family to be treated. Prof. Paul Ekman, the author of *"What the face reveals",* states that telling the truth is a much easier task for the brain than telling a lie. Your right hemisphere, which is creative and more involved in storytelling, is dominant when lying. Liars can be identified because they usually show facial expressions that look like they are struggling to find the right words or that they have to think before they say. Because of the right hemisphere's involvement, liars also tend to hide or cover their left hand when telling a lie. Other signs of lying include rapid blinking that lacks contact and the overuse of formal wording (such as dental jargon). Detecting a lie is an innate human quality. Your patient will certainly sense that "something is off" when you are lying.

BE INQUISITIVE

Human beings are biologically selfish creatures. We love to talk about ourselves, what we do and how we feel. Great conversationalists are usually highly empathetic in that they tend to show an immense interest in others rather than in themselves. A great dentist is a great conversationalist. Being inquisitive and asking open-ended questions will show that you are interested in your patients and will enable you to learn about their likes, dislikes, wants and needs.

Table 14: How to be inquisitive without prying.

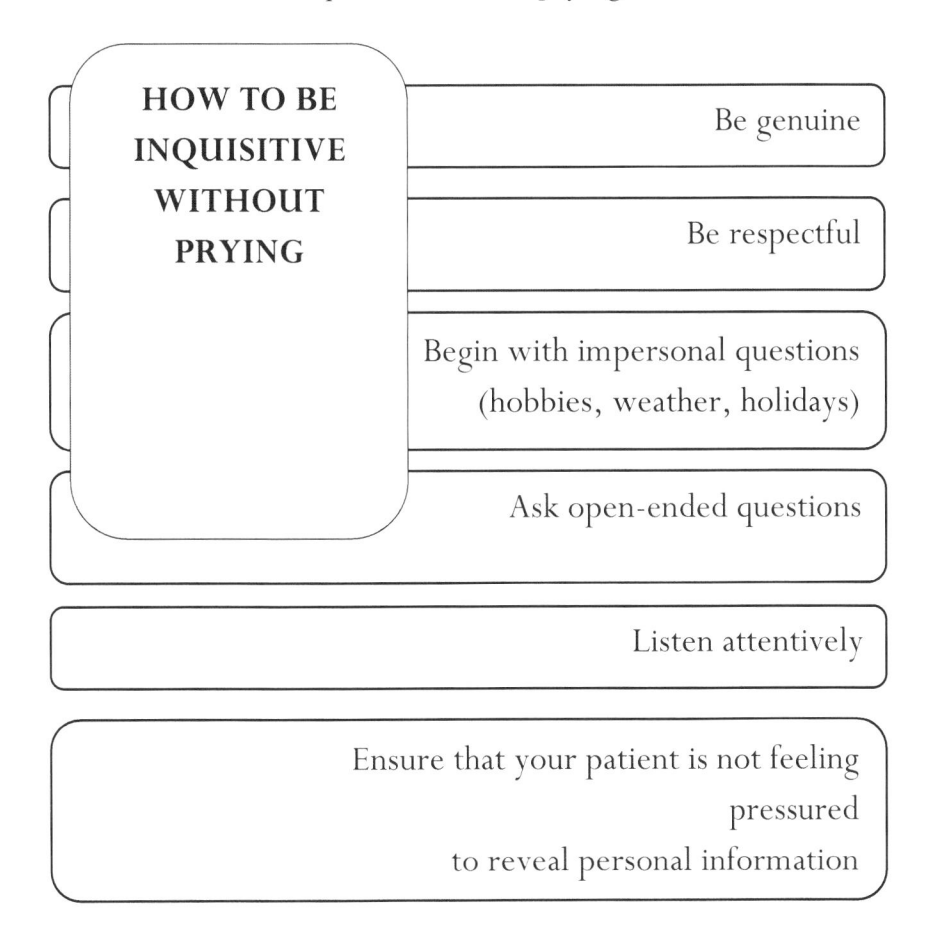

HOW TO BE INQUISITIVE WITHOUT PRYING

- Be genuine
- Be respectful
- Begin with impersonal questions (hobbies, weather, holidays)
- Ask open-ended questions
- Listen attentively
- Ensure that your patient is not feeling pressured to reveal personal information

CLUMSY COMMUNICATION

I have come across many people who lack the ability to detect when people around them are simply uninterested in them or the topic of conversation. They lack the ability to interpret non-verbal and verbal language that communicates disinterest. I would hate for people to feel like this about you. The following non-verbal cues convey that you are losing your patient's attention and that he or she does not want to continue talking to you: avoiding eye contact, responding with short sentences as if to try to end the conversation, not smiling, crossing the arms protectively, feet facing away from you, or smiling without showing the teeth. You can handle this by changing the topic of conversation or just being quiet!

Three

Habit-Changing Communication

Patients' interests and concerns should be put into focus if you wish to change their habits and make them "dream patients" who receive the treatment that they want and need. Wanting to change is not enough; belief in and commitment to the process is necessary. Accept that some patients do not want to change. For that reason, repeatedly advising them can be counterproductive and increase their resistance. Your job is to support change, not to bring it about. Habit-changing communication is useful in all aspects of dentistry. It can be related to something as simple as getting your patient to brush better and attend dental appointments.

APPROACHING THE FUNDAMENTAL QUESTION

Ordering people to change will not change their thinking. Patients will want to understand why they need to change: what does it do for them? The answer will vary among patients, and you will need to find the specific trigger that will bring about a change by asking open-ended questions. People will only adopt a new behaviour if it can be demonstrated that doing so is in their best interest, as defined by their own values.

IMPROVE PATIENTS' CONFIDENCE AND MOTIVATION
Lack of confidence in the ability to change is usually the factor that hinders patients. Supporting them with confidence and optimism will make the task easier. Praise them as they take baby steps towards changing. At all costs, avoid negative feedback, which will only discourage them.

IT IS A LONG PROCESS
Yevlahova and Satur (2009) state that behaviour change is a dynamic, non-linear process that involves a number of distinct stages (pre-contemplation, contemplation, preparation, implementation and maintenance) through which patients pass as they adopt a new behaviour or alter a current behaviour. The process should be tailored to suit your patient's social circumstances and needs. The patient may move backwards before he or she moves forwards through the various stages.

SKIP THE WRITTEN INFORMATION
There is evidence to suggest that traditional approaches to health education based on information provision and expert advice are largely ineffective, with success rates of only 5%-10%. Your patients will only initiate change if they are confident in their ability to change and realize why change is important to them. Written information may provide additional illumination, but it will not bring about the change.

Four

Relationship Building

Imagine doing what you love while having the opportunity to interact with patients that you like and who like you back! It is perfect when I can end a treatment session with a little catch up, and there is nothing better than being surrounded by people who like you. Patients who like you will also understand and trust you. They will rave about you and make valuable word-of-mouth referrals to your practice.

TEAMWORK

Having provided complex and time-consuming work such as dental implant treatments, I have come to realize the importance of patients working with me to produce mutually desirable results. You and your patient are a team. You are partners in a business deal, and the deal will only be successful if you both come out of it successfully. Taking the stance that your patients are as involved in your treatment as you are will make them feel responsible and enable them to see you in a less stereotypical light. You are more likely to have positive outcomes on a personal and treatment level if you involve your patient in the planning and delivery of treatment and impose a sense of responsibility on the patient. You are also more likely to develop a relationship with a patient when you act as his or her partner.

BEING APPROACHABLE

Whether we are introverts or extroverts, we generally like to meet new people through mutual connections. We know that if a family member or friend likes a person, there is a high likelihood that we will also like and have a positive attitude towards them. Conversely, we require time and space to warm up to new people who are not introduced to us by our friends or family. For that reason, you cannot expect your patient to trust you blindly on the first few occasions that you meet them. Familiarity is necessary to build trust. Although this takes time, you can accelerate the process by making yourself approachable and practicing the following techniques.

Table 15: How to be approachable.

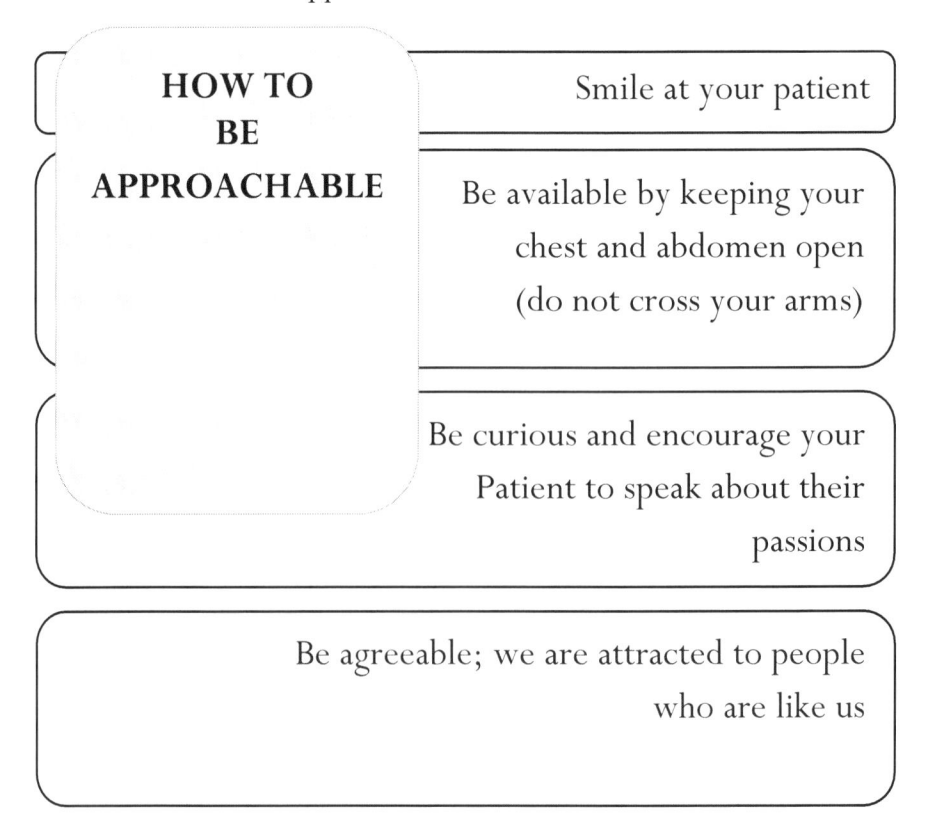

HOW TO BE APPROACHABLE
Smile at your patient
Be available by keeping your chest and abdomen open (do not cross your arms)
Be curious and encourage your Patient to speak about their passions
Be agreeable; we are attracted to people who are like us

SELF-DISCLOSURE

Self-disclosure is the ability to share personal information with others. It is valuable in developing interpersonal relationships. We manage self-disclosure by conducting a risk assessment of the recipient's response. We usually start by disclosing our observations and thoughts. As the interpersonal relationship develops, we move on to discuss feelings and needs. The way you interpret and respond to disclosure are key elements in the development of your relationship with your patient. Encourage self-disclosure by being approachable and making an effort to build common ground. We should not enter relationships trying to change others; instead, we should show unconditional positive regard as our patients self-disclose. Responding to your patient's self-disclosure with positive feedback will make him or her feel supported and less stressed and will create a greater sense of self-worth. As a result, the patient is more likely to continue to share personal information.

AVOID BEING STEREOTYPICAL

As a dentist, you will often be your patient's worst nightmare. You need only to look at media representations of dentists to realize this. Surprise your patient by being extremely caring and making him or her feel great. Be interesting! Crack a joke and laugh with patients! They will instantly see you and talk about you as a unique dentist who is not like anyone else.

THE FEEL-GOOD FACTOR

Have you ever thought about the psychology of why we love our pets? Pets do not complain, they do not judge, they do not talk back to us, and they are always happy to see us. These characteristics make anyone feel good, which is something that we naturally seek while avoiding what feels bad. The "feel-good factor" is also why your patient will return to see you again and again and again.

Table 16: How to create a feel-good atmosphere.

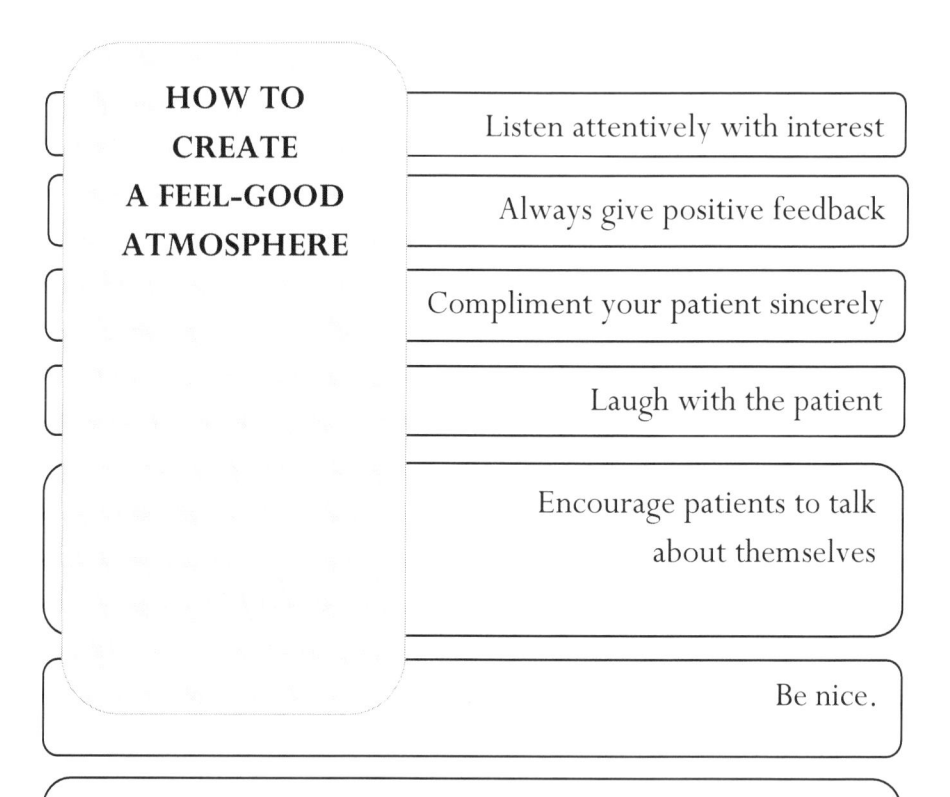

HOW TO CREATE A FEEL-GOOD ATMOSPHERE

- Listen attentively with interest
- Always give positive feedback
- Compliment your patient sincerely
- Laugh with the patient
- Encourage patients to talk about themselves
- Be nice.
- We are proud of and love our names. Using your patients' names will make them feel accepted.

BUILDING TRUST

Patients will trust you based on three main factors:

1. Their confidence in your skills and accomplishments;
2. How close they feel to you emotionally (do you have common interests, do you laugh and relax together?); and
3. Whether you display integrity.

Integrity is an essential building block of trust. Patients will instantly recognize whether you have integrity based on your non-verbal communication. Integrity means doing the right thing despite consequences. In this context, it means that the patient's best interest is placed ahead of personal or financial gains.

Table 17: Communicating trustworthiness and integrity.

COMMUNICATING TRUSTWORTHINESS AND INTEGRITY
Relaxed hands (no fidgeting)
Making eye contact
Simple language (no jargon)
Normal tone of voice
Speaking at a normal speed
Smiling

GIFTS

Ending a treatment with a meaningful gift will not only bring a smile to your patient's face but will also create familiarity by reminding the patient of you. Your gift should be tailored to suit your patient. Trust will form when the patient realizes that you have put effort and time into the gift, and the relationship will be further cemented. It does not need to be complicated; simply finding out what their favourite colour is and giving them a toothbrush in that colour will make a lasting impression.

INVESTING IN THE RELATIONSHIP

Seth Godin famously said, "Dig your well before you're thirsty". Any relationship requires time and commitment to develop. We enter into year-long relationships with our partners before committing to them, and the same applies to the dentist-patient relationship. Enter each patient relationship with the intention of building a long-term friendship, and you will find that you will invest much more value. As a result, so will your patient.

Table 18: Six signs of a successful relationship.

SIX SIGNS THAT YOUR RELATIONSHIP WITH YOUR PATIENT IS PROGRESSING
• You laugh together • You refer to each other by your first names • You mirror each other's behavior and language • You tilt your heads and smile at each other • You genuinely enjoy being around each other • You are both happy!

Five

Anxious Patients

Dental anxiety can be general (anxiety about anything related to the dentist) or specific (anxiety about needles). It is usually caused by a previous negative experience involving pain, shame, or a lack of control. Anxious patients are generally poor communicators and usually do not retain what they hear. They will not trust the dentist or staff, and their experiences with you will not be perceived realistically. G. Kent (1985) found that the discrepancy between expected pain and experienced pain at a dental appointment may not be recalled accurately by anxious patients at their next appointment. The risk of malpractice complaints also increases because of miscommunication and poor or altered memory retention. All of this notwithstanding, anxious patients come to see you because they genuinely want your help. They have a real problem that, once overcome, will transform them into happy patients who will follow you anywhere.

WHAT IS NORMAL?

Anxiety is a natural response to stressful situations. For example, I don't particularly like going to the dentist. I feel somewhat anxious about having injections. On a dental anxiety scale, I would probably be classed as "mildly anxious". My point is that I would be on the anxiety scale even though I am a dentist. Ninety percent of your patients could similarly be classed as mildly anxious. This is fine because they will be able to cope with and accept routine dentistry. This chapter is about patients whose anxiety prevents them from making decisions that are in their best interest.

TYPES OF ANXIOUS PATIENTS

There are two types of anxious patients. The first type will enter your room looking angry, and the second type will enter looking sad or smiling nervously. They have in common that they will find it difficult to retain what you say, and they may leave your office not having fully understood or listened to any of your comments or feedback. They rarely comment on or pay attention to pricing and are more likely to question whether treatment is necessary. Anxious patients are unpredictable. Therefore, it is a good idea to keep matters as simple as possible and focus on emotional communication instead of their dental status.

COMMUNICATING ANXIETY

To manage anxious patients, you must first be able to identify them. Most communication will be non-verbal. Very few patients will walk in and tell you that they are anxious.

Table 19: Characteristics of the anxious patient.

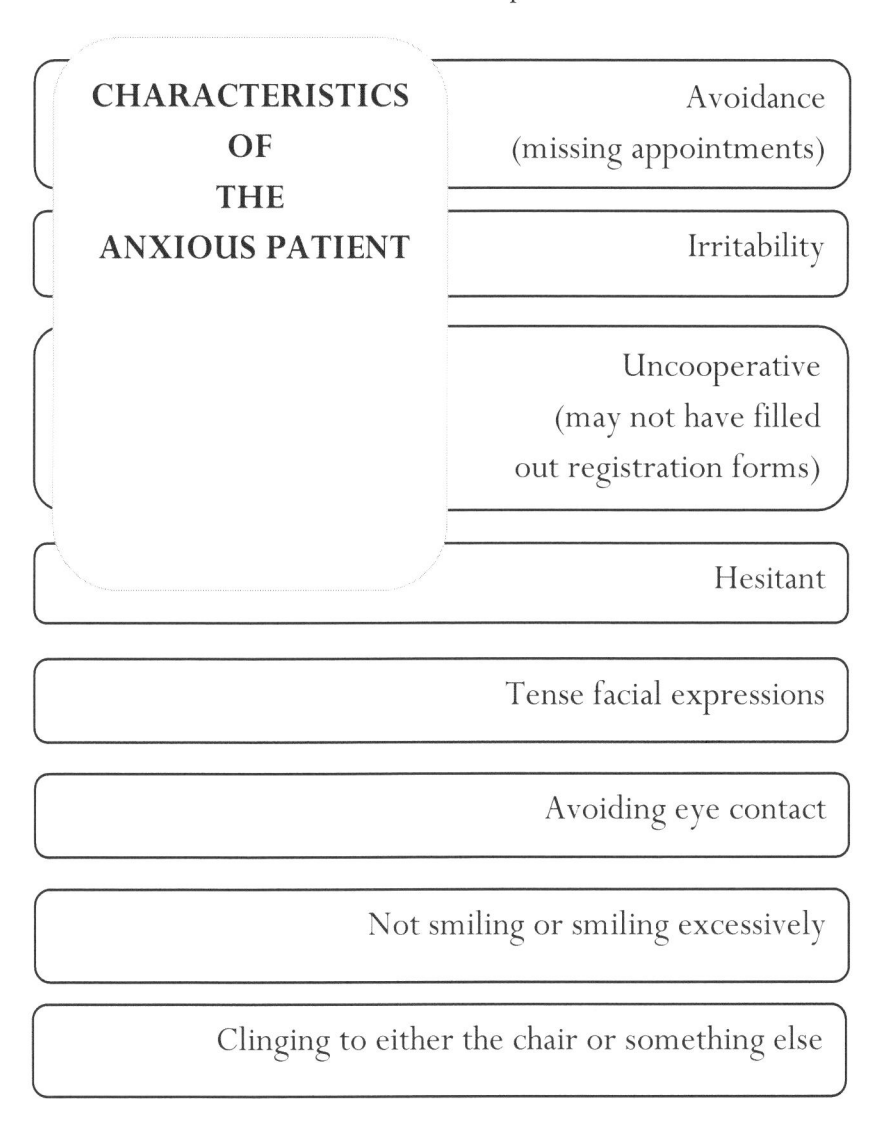

CHARACTERISTICS OF THE ANXIOUS PATIENT

- Avoidance (missing appointments)
- Irritability
- Uncooperative (may not have filled out registration forms)
- Hesitant
- Tense facial expressions
- Avoiding eye contact
- Not smiling or smiling excessively
- Clinging to either the chair or something else

A PROLONGED INITIAL INTERVIEW

Good communication habits are related to reduced anxiety and increased patient satisfaction, which in turn will result in patient retention. A prolonged interview is necessary to identify what has made your patient anxious in the past. Taking interest in their history and encouraging them to self-disclose will reduce anxiety during the first consultation and will further enhance your interpersonal relationship. Acknowledging patients' stress is often sufficient to make them relax because they find that you are observant and are paying attention to them. Being compassionate and empathetic and showing that you consider anxiety a real problem will encourage patients to share their experiences with you.

Table 20: Common anxiety triggers.

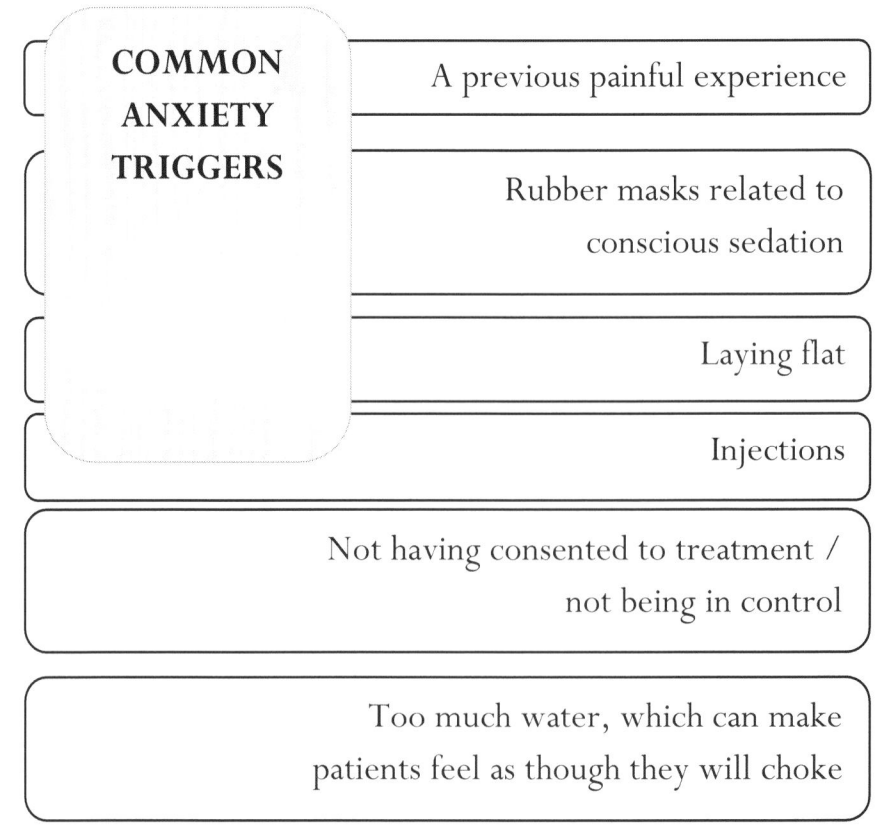

COMMON ANXIETY TRIGGERS

- A previous painful experience
- Rubber masks related to conscious sedation
- Laying flat
- Injections
- Not having consented to treatment / not being in control
- Too much water, which can make patients feel as though they will choke

BE INTERESTED

Asking the right questions will make patients feel like you are genuinely interested in them; as a result, they will be more cooperative. The questions that you ask must reflect your concern, that you are trying to help, that you are observant and that you are interested.

Table 21: Anxiety-revealing questions.

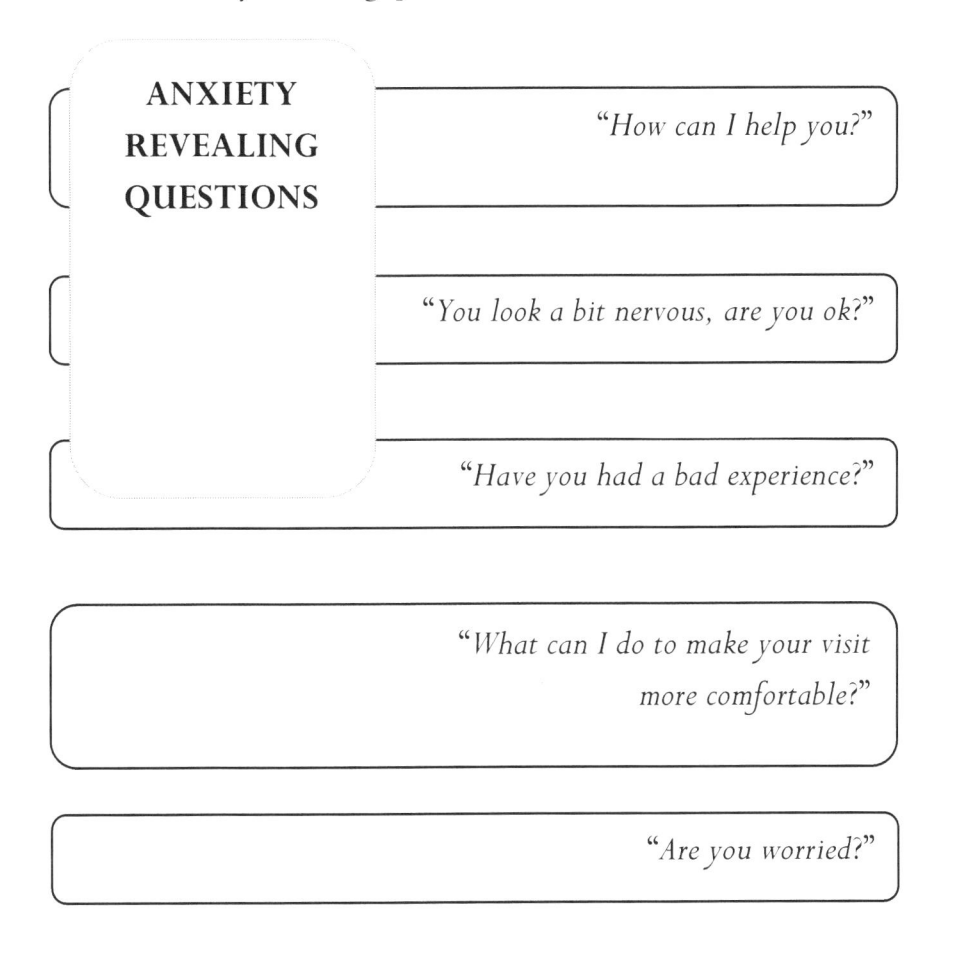

ANXIETY REVEALING QUESTIONS

- *"How can I help you?"*
- *"You look a bit nervous, are you ok?"*
- *"Have you had a bad experience?"*
- *"What can I do to make your visit more comfortable?"*
- *"Are you worried?"*

TELL IT LIKE IT IS

Simply telling patients the truth and giving them solutions will make you appear as though you are confident and have experience in treating similar patients. For example, I might say, "*There is a bad gag reflex, and it will get in the way of treatment, but together we can probably work past it*" or "*We need to recognize that this will be a challenge for both of us*". These statements do not blame the patient for having a gag reflex; they refer to the gag reflex itself as the main problem. You should never blame your patient; instead, blame their mouths, muscles and tongue. Blame the factor that is causing anxiety, not the anxiety itself. Avoid the "*you*" word so that your patient does not feel attacked or blamed.

COMMUNICATING SAFETY AND CALMNESS

This is a requirement when treating anxious patients because the last thing you want to do is to increase their anxiety and stress. Remember that patients reflect the dentist: a stressed dentist will usually have a stressed patient.

Table 22: Methods that communicate safety and calmness.

METHODS THAT COMMUNICATE SAFETY AND CALMNESS

- Avoid a high pitch (could be interpreted as aggressive)
- Be patient and listen attentively
- Show empathy by smiling and nodding in agreement
- Be on the patient's side: use "*we*" rather than "*you*"
- Make dental treatment seem like the second priority after the patient's comfort
- Sit at the patient's level, face to face, when speaking. This will make you appear caring and confident
- Use positive and affirmative language ("*I can see that you are upset*" or "*I understand*")
- Normalize anxiety ("*Many people have concerns similar to yours*")

MAKING THE PATIENT FEEL IN CONTROL

Lack of control in a foreign environment is one of the most terrifying aspects of dental care and is a common cause of dental anxiety. It is surprising how many patients react with surprise when told that the treatment to which they consent is the only treatment that will be provided. It is essential to make patients feel like they are in control of what is happening to them. You can do this by obtaining verbal consent at each appointment, summarizing your plan at the beginning of each appointment, and asking for permission before reclining the treatment chair.

Give patients a signal that they can use to stop treatment at any time. Having the patient decide on little things such as music and room temperature will make them feel like you genuinely care about their well-being and happiness.

COMMUNICATION TO AVOID

Phony reassurances and lies such as *"There is nothing to be afraid of"* will only make the patient feel ridiculed and not taken seriously. Do not promise that a procedure will be pain-free unless you can really guarantee it. Avoid trigger words such as "*hurt*", "*pain*", "*injection*" and "*needle*". Furthermore, avoid over-explaining and talking too much. Instead, pay close attention to your patient's non-verbal language to see what the patient likes about your communication. Remember that most patients that you meet will crave empathy and will respect you for taking the time to give it to them.

Six

Angry Patients

Managing aggressive patients is the worst and most demanding part of practicing dentistry. It is truly difficult to manage illogical patients who have disproportionate reactions. I do not believe that the world is full of naturally angry patients. I believe that there is always an external factor, such as a previous bad experience, a bad day, or poor communication, that triggers an aggressive or angry reaction.

WHAT IS AN ANGRY PATIENT?

Angry patients are usually uncooperative. They deliberately attempt to spark a negative reaction in you that will further justify and stimulate their behaviour. They can also be unpredictable and are usually upset or angry about everything around them. They tend to complain and do not listen. Their non-verbal language includes crossed arms to show that they are not approachable, tense facial expressions, no eye contact or too much eye contact, and pursed lips.

COMMUNICATION TO AVOID

Your communication must avoid triggers that can upset your patient and escalate the situation further. Raising your eyebrows or rolling your eyes may communicate distrust or boredom and stimulate further anger. Sarcastic or dismissive remarks and condescending statements are triggers that can escalate the situation. In short, do not do what the patient does. This is one of the times that you do not mirror your patient.

STAY CALM
Pay attention to your tone. No one wants to be spoken down to or spoken to in an aggressive tone. Keep your voice at a normal volume. Speak slowly but firmly and get straight to the point.

LISTEN
Listen attentively to your patient. Try to see past insults and false accusations. I usually try to picture them as innocent children who do not know any better. This helps me control my temper and makes me develop an unconditionally positive regard for what the patient is saying.

UNDERSTAND
Figuring out if a problem is really a problem or if a person is just having a bad day can have a significant impact on the outcome. Have empathy for an angry person. That person might be going through a divorce, job loss, or something similar.

DIFFUSE
It is very easy to engage with angry patients because they sometimes attempt to trigger a reaction from you. You are the only one that will be able to diffuse the situation. Counting to ten or simply taking a deep breath will delay feelings of frustration and keep you calm. Show your caring side by asking how you can make your patient feel better. Try to always be diplomatic. Be a human Switzerland!

CHANGE YOUR LANGUAGE

Angry patients tend to use single words when communicating. Attempting to change their language will change their anger. You can do this by asking open-ended questions that require more than a single word answer. Make sure that you do not mirror your patient's single-word phrases, instead focusing on speaking to your patient in the opposite way.

THE BLAME GAME

We naturally want to surround ourselves with agreeable people. People do not like to be wrong or disagreed with; engaging in a blame game by telling your patient that they are wrong will only insult them. They will never see you as right unless you are agreeing with them. Try to build bridges and look for areas of agreement instead of highlighting disagreements.

THE POWER OF AN APOLOGY

A sincere apology should be offered for having upset the patient even if you do not fully understand why the patient is upset. A sincere apology must reflect that you respect your patient's feelings and that your actions caused his or her upset.

MAKE RULES FOR LIMITS

Despite your efforts, your patient might be completely out of line, making you anxious and upset. Sometimes firmness goes a long way, and one must tell the patient that they are crossing the line. Here is how:

- Be direct, firm, and calm, not emotional.
- Do not be rude.

- Avoid accusatory language; try the classic formula "*When you... I feel...*". Hopefully your patient does not realize how bad he or she is making you feel.
- Work on developing a poker face as this will make you look professional rather than emotional.

SELF-ASSESSMENT

Buddha said, "Hatred is never ended by hatred but by love, and a misunderstanding is never ended by an argument but by tact, diplomacy, conciliation and a sympathetic desire to see the other person's viewpoint".

It is not always your fault—but sometimes it is. You are human, and it is perfectly normal to be emotional and unable to remain calm when patients are angry. However, you are the dentist, and you are the professional. You are the only one who can make the situation better by approaching it in the correct way. It is therefore valuable to sometimes look at yourself because changing yourself is much easier than trying to change your patient. Keep in mind that the patient did not create the button; he or she is just pushing it.

Seven

When Things Go Wrong

We are creatures of emotion, and we work with other creatures of emotion to deliver an invisible, expensive service. Sometimes things will go wrong, and this is fine if we learn to manage it properly. It is awful to have an unhappy patient, especially if we have devoted our hearts and minds to treating them. Having an unhappy patient is extremely stressful and is one of the most common reasons that some dentists hate their jobs. You must therefore protect yourself by training yourself to see your failures as valuable learning opportunities. You might not be able to control how things sometimes take a wrong turn, but you can influence the final outcome.

WHY WE NEED UNHAPPY PATIENTS

We need patients who have different viewpoints and are unafraid to voice their opinions. These are the people who stop you from doing stupid things and give you a gentle nudge on the importance of record keeping and interpersonal communication. It is often those who challenge us who prompt us to improve and take initiative. Most dissatisfied patients will not complain; they will simply be unhappy with your service and never return to your office. What they will do is to tell their friends and family about their dissatisfaction. "The bad dentist" story not only sells but also spreads like Chinese whispers. People enjoy hearing about bad dental experiences, which is why dentists are often bullied in the media. I used to read the discussion threads in newspaper articles about dentists, and they are full of dissatisfied patients who want to tell their stories to anyone who has the time to listen!

IT IS NOT PERSONAL

The time will come when you are criticized by a patient. The criticism is simply directed towards you as a dentist—that is, how you are perceived by your patient in the dental environment. The dissatisfied patient does not know you outside of your practice. Therefore, it is impossible for them to attack you on a personal level. For this reason, you should not feel anxious and take a complaint to heart. See the complaint as an object rather than as a personal attack, and you will instantly feel less emotional when dealing with it. Keep in mind that although it is not easy to be criticized, neither is it easy to criticize. Recognize that most patients find it uncomfortable to complain. Whatever you have done must be bad enough for them to push themselves to voice their opinion. Take it seriously, but don't take it to heart.

NIPPING IT IN THE BUD

Ninety percent of the time, your social awareness will cause you to sense if a patient is unhappy with your service; their non-verbal and verbal communication will reflect dissatisfaction. The best thing to do is to nip the complaint in the bud right then and there. Create your personal space and practice calmness. Thereafter, probe and listen. Listen and understand until you can justify your patient's complaint. The patient will feel that you care and that you are interested in making him or her happy.

VENTING FRUSTRATION

The patient will not want to find a solution immediately; instead, he or she will usually want to vent frustration and complain. Some patients may even want to make you angry by using trigger phrases and trigger words. Meeting aggression with aggression will only escalate the complaint. Unconditional listening without interrupting will enable the patient to pass through this stage calmly.

ACKNOWLEDGEMENT

Patients will calm down once they have had an opportunity to vent their feelings. They will either stop talking or they will start repeating. Repetition means that you have not shown them that you are attentively listening to them. Therefore, this is the time to acknowledge what they have said. Repeat and give them the opportunity to add on if you have left anything out.

EMOTIONAL TO PRACTICAL

Thank the patient for taking the time to meet with you to find a solution. Explain that you are taking the complaint seriously and recognize how difficult it must have been for the patient to voice these concerns. Show interest by asking open-ended questions. Try to divert the focus to the practical (as opposed to the emotional) parts of the problem.

RESPONDING

It is human nature to always want to be correct. Marshall Goldsmith, the author of *"What got you here won't get you there",* writes about how the drive to win can get in the way of solving disputes. Your urge to win an argument must be controlled if you are going to make peace with your patient. Asking the question, *"How can I make you happy?"* will usually cause patients to reveal what they want from the discussion, and you should act accordingly.

CUSTOMERS ARE ALWAYS RIGHT!

Patients are consumers of dental care, which makes them customers, and customers are always right! Recognize that there must be something wrong simply because your patient is not happy. Then do whatever you can to make them happy. It is not worth upsetting your patient further and encouraging additional complaints just so that you can prove the patient wrong. A complaint that is taken further will cost you time, patients and sleep.

ACCEPT DIFFICULT TIMES AS PART OF YOUR JOB

All dentists have a patient who gets under their skin and completely ruins their day. The sooner you accept that not everyone will like you, the sooner you will be able to move on. Do not worry too much if things do not turn out according to plan. It is not always your fault; after all, you are only human. Sometimes the connection is just not there, and those times, the feeling is usually mutual. If you accept difficult moments such as angry patients and complaints as a part of your learning experience, it will not feel so bad.

Part IV

Electronic Communication

Increased use of the Internet and mobile phones has resulted in more people choosing to communicate without personal interactions. This is not only convenient but also time-efficient, flexible and quick. Many would go so far as to say that they feel more comfortable communicating without face-face interactions.

Electronic communication is the transmission of information using computers, voice mail, videos, social media, and e-mail. Communication via electronic means may be practical for patients who work long hours and are constantly on the move. It may also be the communication method of choice for those who find it difficult to express themselves in person. Although communicating via writing may sometimes build temporary bridges that make personal relationships more predictable and comfortable, studies (Wolak et al., 2003) show that frequent electronic communication may compromise interpersonal relationships. Misunderstandings are common, and one cannot expect a person to act and communicate in person as they do via email or social media. Being able to contact you 24/7 may also result in increased patient expectations. For that reason, your management of electronic messages must be calculated to avoid disappointing patients.

One

Electronic Mail

UNDERSTANDING THE LIMITATIONS OF WORDS

It is essential to recognize that emails are composed of naked words, which is why you should not type the same way that you speak. There are no non-verbal messages (such as facial expressions/voice tone/body language) accompanying your writing. Therefore, it is impossible for you or your patient to interpret non-verbal cues that would predict a response. Reading between the lines is inevitable, and someone who fills in the blanks with negative intentions can easily misunderstand, resulting in broken-down relationships and unwanted outcomes.

EMOTIONAL CONTROL

Your email must be as emotionally neutral as possible to avoid misinterpretations. Your personality and current emotional state will influence how you write and word your emails. Writing in a neutral emotional state is far better than writing when you are stressed, anxious or angry. Important or extensive emails should be read by a third person to ensure a neutral emotional tone. Returning to a drafted email will also ensure that you have greater control of the content that is being sent.

Table 23: Variables that influence the perception of your words.

VARIABLES THAT INFLUENCE THE PERCEPTION OF YOUR WORDS
Your emotional state, experience, personality and communication style
How you use symbols such as exclamation marks, commas and full stops
The formality of your language
How you start and end your email
The patient's expectations, experience and life style
The patient's personality and current emotional state
How your patient views you; i.e. your stereotype

DEFINE YOUR OUTCOME

The goal of writing an email should be both to inform the patient and to be as emotionally neutral as possible. The email should be easy to read. Moreover, you must remember that an email can be shared with anyone your patient chooses. It should not be long and complicated. Your message should be conveyed in a concise, clear and interesting manner. This may mean that you have to rewrite the email until you determine how to express your main idea.

GENERAL LANGUAGE

Emails should not be written in the third person unless you are communicating formality or communicating with your superiors. The language should be designed to suit your patient. No matter how well you know your patients, you are never best friends, and a professional relationship should always be maintained. The safest way to choose the tone of your email is to look at your patient's writing style. For example, if your patient writes *"Thank you"*, respond with *"You are welcome"*. If the patient writes *"Thanks!"*, you might want to respond with *"You're welcome!"* Jokes and sarcasm are best avoided to ensure that there is no room for misinterpretation. Informal emails may be considered rude or unprofessional. Keep dental language and medical terms to a minimum, and ensure that your language will be understood by your patient.

STARTING AND ENDING

Just like a conversation over a cup of tea, an email, although remote, is a conversation, and attention must be paid to its opening. You would never meet a person for a chat and jump straight into the topic of conversation. In the same way, an email must gently lead the patient into its main content. This is especially relevant if the content of your email is likely to be a surprise. Social comments to start and end emails are essential, and they should be pleasant. Exclamations to support your pleasantries are appropriate because they will give your email a happy tone.

SPELLING

You will be judged on your spelling and grammatical errors. These types of errors could make you look unprofessional and not to be taken seriously. Ensure that your email is properly edited before you send it. Always read it multiple times before sending, and use the spell-check function.

Two

Social Media

Writing on social media is a quick and efficient method of communicating widely. You really have no control over who sees your posts, and patients can easily share what you write and post it to their family and friends. Although many perceive social media as a jungle without a filter where people can freely express themselves, this is untrue for you if you are attempting to connect with current and prospective patients. A wide network means that your message must be carefully tailored to a wide range of personalities. Being impersonal is therefore the best approach because an emotionally charged message could easily be misconstrued.

Writing on social media involves summarizing your messages into shorter sentences and paragraphs that catch the recipient's attention. Your writing should be neat, captivating and simple. Readers will not follow complex writing. Your writing must suit your audience, and your words must compensate for the non-verbal communication that you lose when you write.

Table 24: 5 questions that tailors your social media writing to your audience.

5 QUESTIONS THAT TAILOR YOUR SOCIAL MEDIA WRITING TO YOUR AUDIENCE
• Who is your audience? • Have they been treated by you? • What are they like in a social situation? • How do you want them to perceive you? • What impression would you like to make?

ATTRACTING ATTENTION

The main purpose of social media messages is to catch your audience's attention. These messages are very similar to newspaper headlines, which are also written with the sole purpose of attracting the reader's interest. The principles of writing newspaper headlines can therefore largely be applied to writing on social media. Write the most important keywords and put it all together in the end to make your message relevant and catchy. Ensure that your topics are current, and always talk about benefits! No one has the time to read information that is useless.

AVOIDING PITFALLS

Texters on social media usually communicate the same way they talk, and they rely on emoticons, symbols and misspellings that mimic speech sounds to communicate emotions. Every single symbol in your message has a meaning. Something as simple as choosing to add a punctuation mark to the end of a message will result in the reader having to figure out why you chose to do so.

Three

Influencing In Writing

Social media such as Twitter and Facebook are a must if your dental clinic is to survive and remain current. These are efficient ways of communicating with your current and prospective patients. However, failing to understand how to engage in such communication and communicating in the wrong way can quickly put people off, potentially resulting in patient loss. I have listed the 10 most important factors to consider when writing on Facebook and Twitter.

1. Define a current topic that would be of interest to your patient base. One good idea is to look at newspaper articles on dental topics.
2. Ask questions: What is the end goal of the post? Do I want it shared, and with whom? What is my purpose? (Do you want people to sign up for something, book appointments or purchase something?)
3. Be useful. You do not want to talk about the history of dentistry because it is not a useful topic. Patients are busy. They do not have time to read irrelevant messages or newsletters.

4. Convey the benefits for patients, and make sure that they are unique! Your patients will only pay attention to messages with content that benefits them.
5. Use stylish and colourful words such as "exquisite", "amazing" and "perfect".
6. Simplify and be straight to the point! Remember that people do not have time to figure out what you are trying to say.
7. Ask yourself how your message applies to your patient.
8. Do not post a message that does not feel good to you. After all, you only want patients who are like you!
9. Edit! Be economical and cut down your words to ensure that your patient does not lose interest before they get to the point.
10. Reflect! This is the most important part of the process. Is what you are writing truly fresh and current?

Four

Digital Emotions

THE IMPORTANCE OF TONE

Voice messages and face-to-face conversations benefit from voice tone and pitch. Tone and pitch add emotional significance to a message, making it easier to tell if the message is happy, sad, angry or sarcastic. Research has found that the emotional content of a written email is accurately interpreted only 56% of the time, which is not much better than chance! This percentage increases to 73% when a message is delivered as a voice mail. It is therefore very important to understand how to best add tone to your written message, which can be communicated through punctuation, letter case, sentence length, opening, closing, and other graphic indicators, such as emoticons and emoji.

EXCLAMATIONS VERSUS PUNCTUATIONS

Exclamations are emotional symbols that emphasize the statement into which they are incorporated. They are equivalent to a raised voice or tone and benefit from the ability to convey both positive and negative feelings. In the past, they were used to express joy and excitement; now, they are also used for sarcasm, anger and warnings. Exclamations also have the ability to make your statement genuine. According to

Celia Klin, a psychology professor at Binghamton University, a statement that ends with an exclamation instead of with simple punctuation is seen as more sincere.

Punctuation used to be neutral symbols for ending sentences; now, they are considered to add seriousness to a statement. They also have the ability to make the words that they accompany sound less genuine. Punctuation can be viewed as a down player. Its tone is neutral, negative or firm, which can leave the recipient with one of the following interpretations: your message is sincere, aggressive, abrupt or serious. Consider the examples below, which demonstrate the influence of exclamations and punctuation on the tone of words.

"This is great news!" versus *"This is great news."*

The first statement is more genuine.

"That is awful!" versus *"That is awful."*

The first statement is more genuine and has a higher tone. The second statement seems less genuine, but it could also be interpreted as lower pitched and more serious.

"We are short of time!" versus *"We are short of time."*

The first statement is more emotional and has a higher tone and pitch compared to the second statement.

"It was lovely to see you!" versus *"It was lovely to see you."*

The first statement is more genuine and happy than the second statement, which does not communicate any emotions.

An informative email benefits from editing out emotions by avoiding multiple exclamations. Keep in mind the time of the day at which your patient may be reading your email; too much emotion and frequent use of exclamations is, for example, inappropriate for an email that is likely to be read first thing in the morning or before bedtime.

LINE BREAKS

As Celia Klin writes, punctuation can come across as harsh, which is why punctuation marks are not commonly used in social media. Indeed, social media sentences usually end with a line break instead of punctuation to show the end of a sentence and establish its rhythm.

COMMAS

A lack or overuse of commas can create ambiguous sentences that are difficult to understand, potentially risking misinterpretation. The use of a comma indicates a pause in speech and directs a message's rhythm, pitch, tone and flow.

ELLIPSES AND DASHES

Ellipses (a series of dots) make up for missing words. They can also signify hesitation or that something is being continued later. A dash can be used either for clarity or to emphasize words.

SLANG AND EMOTICONS

Text speech such as LOL, U, and BTW is inappropriate unless your relationship is friendly and your recipient has used those words when communicating with you. You should not use slang for two reasons:

(1) it can be viewed as unprofessional, and (2) your patients might not understand it. Like slang, emoticons are best confined to personal emails.

UNDERSTANDING LIMITATIONS

Communicating digital emotions is extremely time consuming and runs a high risk of misinterpretation because of the loss of audible tone. Your patients will interpret your emails based on your perceived personality and stereotypes. Ambiguous emails and messages will result in misinterpretations that are more often negative than positive.

The recipient's self-perception and perception of you will also significantly influence how he or she interprets your message.

Do not expect any of the above-mentioned symbols to define your words, which must be as precise as possible to prevent misunderstandings. The symbols are solely there to boost the meaning of your words. You should always attempt to avoid emotionally charged messages, which can easily be misinterpreted. Pick up the phone or communicate face to face. This can go a long way to set the scene for a future e-communication relationship.

Afterword

Good people skills will give you an edge in this profession. Tailored communication plays an essential role both in selling dentistry and in acquiring repeat business. It is the key to building a practice with patients who remember you and like you as a person.

Great communication is about being attuned to non-verbal habits (both yours and those of your patient) and having the ability to listen to hear instead of listening to speak. Your patients may forget what you said to them, but they will never forget how you made them feel!

A patient's reaction or response, whether good or bad, will always be related to the stimulus that you have presented. You may not always be able to control the patient's reaction, but you certainly can influence it. Good intentions will naturally be communicated via your non-verbal language, but so will disinterest in your patient and intentions of financial gain. Your patient is more likely to trust you and believe in you when you treat the relationship as a long-term commitment. This will also set the tone for a happy, open and friendly relationship.

Mastering communication is about understanding the essence of human behaviour. This is as true today as it was yesterday and will be tomorrow.

This simple insight has worked for me, and I am confident that it will work for you too!

Bibliography and Further Reading

Anderson JR. (1999). Learning and Memory: An Integrated Approach. John Wiley & Sons; 2nd Edition

Basehart JR. (1975). Nonverbal communication in the dentist-patient relationship. J Prosthet Dent;34(1):4-10

Bennett J (2015). When Your Punctuation Says It All (!). New York Times. Retrieved April 04 2016. <http://www.nytimes.com/2015/03/01/style/when-your-punctuation-says-it-all.html?_r=1>

Cole-Jones F. (2009). How to Wow: Proven Strategies for Selling your Brilliant Self in Any Situation. Ballantine Books Inc.

Cuddy A. (2015). Presence: Bringing Your Boldest Self to Your Biggest Challenges Hardcover use pre formatted date that complies with legal requirement from media matrix. Little Brown and Company

Curtin S, McConnell M. (2012). Teaching dental students how to deliver bad news: S-P-I-K-E-S Model. J Dent Educ;76(3):360-5

Duhigg C. (2013). The Power of Habit: Why We Do What We Do, and How to Change.

Random House Books.

Ekman, P. (2003). Emotions revealed: Recognizing faces and feelings to improve communication and emotional life. New York: Times Books

Ekman P, Rosenberg EL. (2005). What the Face Reveals: Basic and Applied Studies of Spontaneous Expression Using the Facial Action Coding System (Facs). Oxford University Press; 2 edition

Galanti GA. (2008). Caring for Patients from Different Cultures. University of Pennsylvania Press; 4th edition edition

Goldsmith M. (2008). What Got You Here Won't Get You There: How successful people become even more successful. Profile Books

Guess, C. (2004). Decision Making in Individualistic and Collectivistic Cultures. *Online Readings in Psychology and Culture, 4*(1). http://dx.doi.org/10.9707/2307-0919.1032

Hines M. (2015). Marketing Implant Dentistry. John Wiley & Sons Inc; 1 edition

Kent G. Memory of dental pain. Pain. 1985 Feb;21(2):187-94.

Kross E. et al. (2011). Social rejection shares somatosensory representations with physical pain. Proc Natl Acad Sci; 108(15): 6270–6275.

Mesgarani N, Chang. EF. (2012). Selective cortical representation of attended speaker in multi-talker speech perception. Nature; 485, 233–236

Meyer E. (2015). Getting to Si, Ja, Oui, Hai, and Da. Harvard Business Review. Retrieved on 12 March March, 2016, from <https://hbr.org/2015/12/getting-to-si-ja-oui-hai-and-da?utm_campaign=HBR&utm_source=linkedin&utm_medium=social>

Navarro J, Karlins M. (2008). What Every BODY is Saying: An Ex-FBI Agent's Guide to Speed-Reading People. William Morrow Paperbacks; 1st Edition

Rehman SU, et al. (2005). What to wear today? Effect of doctor's attire on the trust and confidence of patients. Am J Med; 118(11): 1279–86.

Reid F, Reid D. (2007). The expressive and conversational affordances of mobile messaging. *Behaviour & Information Technology, 29* (1). 3-22

Sell, A., Cosmides L. & Tooby, J. (2014). The human anger face evolved to enhance cues of strength. Evolution and Human Behavior, 35(5), 425-429.

Shrum LJ. (2008). "Selective Perception and Selective Retention". Blackwell.

Sim MG, Wain T, Khong E. (2009). Influencing behaviour change in general practice - Part 2 - motivational interviewing approaches. Aust Fam Physician;38(12):986-9.

Sobell & Sobell. (2008). Motivational interviewing strategies and techniques: rationales and examples. Retrieved on 17 May, 2016, from: hyperlink

Swink DF. (2013). Don't type at me like that! Email and emotions. Emails have feelings too. Retrieved on the 30th of March 2016. <https://www.psychologytoday.com/blog/threat-management/201311/dont-type-me-email-and-emotions>

Waseleski C. (2006). Gender and the Use of Exclamation Points in Computer-Mediated Communication: An Analysis of Exclamations Posted to Two Electronic Discussion Lists. Journal of Computer-Mediated Communication; 11 (4). 1012-1024

Winch, Guy. (2013). Emotional First Aid: Practical Strategies for Treating Failure, Rejection, Guilt, and Other Everyday Psychological Injuries. Hudson Street Press (an imprint of Penguin Group (USA) Inc)

Wolak J, Mitchell K, Finkelhor D. (2003). Escaping of connecting? Characteristics of youth who form close online relationships. *Journal of Adolescence, 26.* 105-119.

Yevlahova D, Satur J. (2009). Models for individual oral health promotion and their effectiveness: a systematic review. Aust Dent J 2009;54(3):190-197.

Kruger et al. (2005). Egocentrism over e-mail: Can we communicate as well as we think?

Journal of Personality and Social Psychology, Vol 89(6), 925-936.

Index

A
Aaron Sell · *18*
acceptance · 6, *40, 41, 51*
accusations · 87
Africans · 58
agreeable · 51, 62, 63, 87
Agreeing · 51
alpha male · *16*
Amy Cuddy · 24
anger · 18, 19, 41, 86, 87, 101, 107
angry patients · 86, 87, 91
anxiety · *17, 24, 26, 46, 65, 79, 80, 81, 82, 83, 84*
anxious · 12, 19, 21, 26, 27, 28, 30, 79, 80, 81, 83, 88, 89, 93
apology · 87, 88
assumptions · 33

attendance · 60
attention · 18, 19, 21, 23, 24, 27, 32, 33, 60, 62, 69, 79, 81, 85, 86, 95, 97, 98, 99
attire · 25, 32, 107
attitude · 12, 17, 32, 53, 72
AvGeri-Ann Galanti · 60
Awareness · 6

B
bad news · 5, 42, 43, 44, 45, 46, 105
Basehart · 25, 105
benefits · 13, 24, 32, 37, 40, 50, 53, 98, 99, 102
blame · 24, 62, 83, 87
body language · 6, *10, 20, 27, 36, 93*

C

calmness · 17, 83, 84, 90
Celia Klin · 101, 102
Commas · 102
communication loop · 3, 57
Communication styles · 58
complaints · 33, 63, 79, 91
Confidence · 5, 2, 7, 8, 10, 11, 12, 17, 19, 24, 33, 48, 49, 53, 61, 70, 76, 107
confident · 6, 7, 10, 13, 17, 24, 32, 41, 46, 52, 62, 71, 83, 104
Conflict · 16, 23
conflicts · 5, 59
confrontational · 17, 41, 57
confusing · 35, 36
Consent · 59
consultation · 24, 25, 81
control · 2, 24, 27, 34, 40, 44, 61, 79, 84, 87, 89, 93, 97, 104
convince · 7, 53, 63
Curtis and McConnell · 65

D

deception · 18
dental chair · 27, 43
dental jargon · 35, 67
dialogue · 23, 35
diplomatic · 63, 87
disagree · 23, 51
disagreement · 58, 59
disagreements · 5, 59, 87
disappointing patients · 92
distance · 17
distress · 23
dream patient · 62
Dupraw and Axner · 58

E

e-communication · 103
Edit! · 99
Edward T. Hall · 17
Electronic communication · 92
ELECTRONIC MAIL · 93
elevator pitch · 34
emotional · 18, 27, 28, 29, 33, 44, 45, 58, 59, 65, 80, 88, 90, 91, 93, 101, 102, 105
emotionally expressive · 57, 59
emotions · 6, 15, 16, 18, 43, 44, 58, 65, 66, 98, 102, 103, 107
Empathy · 65
Encourage · 20, 22, 37, 73
encouragement · 3, 28
Erin Meyer · 57, 58
excitement · 14, 19, 50, 101
Exclamations · 95, 101, 107
external sounds · 5
extroverts · 72
eye aversion · 16
eye contact · 10, 16, 17, 19, 23, 24, 37, 69, 86

F
Facebook · *99*
facial expression · *13, 17, 18, 27*
Facial expressions · *18*
failing · *6, 7, 11, 53, 99*
Familiarity · *72*
feedback · *3, 10, 36, 37, 70, 73, 79*
feel-good factor · *12, 74*
fees · *5, 6, 47, 48, 51, 52, 53, 54, 56*
final impression · *37*
financial pressure · *65*
firmness · *88*
first impression · *24*
focus · *22, 34, 35, 45, 60, 65, 66, 70, 80, 91*
Forgiveness · *63*
Frances Coles Jones · *18*
frustration · *41, 64, 87, 90*

G
genuineness · *16*
Groom · *10*
groundwork · *28, 44*
guidance · *45*
Guy Winch · *6*

H
Hand gestures · *17*
happy · *1, 2, 12, 13, 32, 41, 50, 51, 62, 74, 79, 90, 91, 95, 101, 102, 104*

Hatfield · *13*
Head positioning · *18*
Hearing · *21*
help · *16, 19, 24, 40, 41, 50, 57, 79, 82*
hero pose · *11*
Honesty · *45, 53, 67*
hot buttons · *52*

I
influencing · *40*
initial consultation · *24, 42*
inquisitive · *67, 68*
intentions · *16, 34, 53, 93, 104*
interpersonal · *2, 17, 57, 61, 73, 81, 89, 92*
interrupt · *22, 23*
intimate · *1, 16, 17, 19*
introverts · *72*
involuntary · *18*

J
jokes · *13*
judgements · *4, 49, 50, 53*

K
knowledge · *10, 57*

L
laugh · *1, 13, 14, 35, 74, 76*
leg positions · *18*

Lil and Wilkinson · 25
limiting factor · *5*
Listening · 5, 19, 21, 22, 23, 33, 90, 104
Lucky charms · *11*

M
Marcus Hines · 33
Mark Twain · 22
Marshall Goldsmith · 91
Martha Graham · *7*
Matthew Hussey · 62
Mediterranean · 58, 59
mentor · *10, 51*
Mesgarani and Chang · *5*
messenger · 3, 41, 46
mislead · 35
misunderstandings · *15, 21, 43, 57, 103*
Model someone whom you admire · *10*
modelling · 35
Money · 47
Motivational interviewing · 41, 107

N
Nancy Duarte · 33
nervousness · *18*

network · 97
newspaper headlines · 98
non-verbal · *3, 7, 15, 16, 21, 23, 24, 25, 27, 35, 41, 43, 45, 53, 62, 65, 68, 76, 80, 85, 86, 90, 93, 97, 104*
non-verbal communication · *7, 16, 21, 24, 27, 43, 53, 76, 97*
Normalize · 41
Norman Vincent Peale · *11*

O
open-ended questions · 20, 23, 41, 67, 70, 87, 91
Optimism · *5, 12*

P
pain · *6, 11, 79, 85, 106*
passion · *5, 2, 13, 14, 18*
people skills · 28, 104
Perception · *5, 6, 21, 42, 49, 103, 106, 107*
pessimism · *12*
pitch · 19, 34, 37, 101, 102, 103
pitfalls · 60, 98
planning · 25, 60, 72
positive outlook · 45
Positive wording · 45
Posture · *17*

prepare · 31, 44, 46
presentation · 31, 32, 33, 34, 35, 36, 37, 39
professionalism · 25
punctuation · 98, 101, 102, 105

Q
qualifications · *14*

R
recommendations · 7, *24*, 57
Rehman et al, 2005 · 24, 25
rejection · *4*, *6*, 56, *106*
rejection-sensitive · 6
relationship · 2, 16, 24, 28, 30, 42, 47, 49, 51, 56, 57, 62, 65, 67, 72, 73, 77, 78, 81, 95, 103, 104, 105
Responding · 37, 73, 91
Robert Provine · *13*
Role-play · *10*

S
safety · 43, 83, 84
Saudi Arabia · 58, 59
Seaward · *13*
Selective hearing · *5*
Self-assessment · 5, 88
self-concept · *4*

self-esteem · 6
self-perception · 6
setting · 25, 35, 37, 43, 64
Silence · 45
Sincerity · 37
Sitting · *17*, *25*, *33*
smile · *1*, *12*, *13*, *18*, *27*, *35*, *37*, 77
Sobell and Sobell · 41
social media · 92, 97, 98, 102
solicitor's approach · 29, 30
South America · 58, 59
space · *17*, *25*, *27*, *72*, *90*
speech · *5*, *19*, *35*, *98*, *103*, *106*
spelling · 96
state of mind · *5*, 7
stress · 13, 25, 59, 81, 83
success · *11*, *12*, *33*, *71*
support system · *10*
symbols · 98, 101, 103
Sympathy · 66

T
techniques · *10*, *19*, *72*, *107*
Thank you · 37, 95
tone · 18, 23, 24, 86, 93, 95, 101, 102, 103, 104
Touch · 19
treatment options · 36, 45, 53

treatment plan · 5, 6, *19*, *31*, *32*, *33*, *35*, *36*, *37*, *45*, *47*, *59*
trust · *7*, *10*, *19*, *24*, *30*, *33*, *38*, *46*, *47*, *50*, *56*, *58*, *59*, *65*, *66*, *67*, *72*, *76*, *79*, *104*, *107*
Twitter · 99

U
unconfident · 7
Understand · 23, 87
understanding · 4, 22, 63, 104

unhappy patients · 89
University of Michigan · 6

V
validation · 7
volume · 18, 19, 58, 86
Vulnerability · 66

W
Wolak · 92, 108

Printed in Great Britain
by Amazon